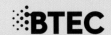

PEARSON
FIRST PERSON ON SCENE

FOR THE 2016 SPECIFICATION
BTEC LEVEL 4 CERTIFICATE AND EXTENDED CERTIFICATE

SECOND EDITION

Adam Gent
Nic Gunn

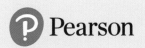

Published by Pearson Education Limited, 80 Strand, London, WC2R 0RL.

http://qualifications.pearson.com/en/qualifications/btec-specialist-and-professional-qualifications/

Text © Pearson Education Limited 2017
Typeset by Cambridge Publishing Management
Original illustrations © Pearson Education Limited 2017
Cover illustration © Pearson Education Limited 2017

The rights of Adam Gent and Nic Gunn to be identified as authors of this work have been asserted by them in accordance with the Copyright, Designs and Patents Act 1988.

First edition published 2004 (reprinted 10 times)
Second edition published 2017

20 19 18 17
10 9 8 7 6 5 4 3 2 1

British Library Cataloguing in Publication Data
A catalogue record for this book is available from the British Library

ISBN 978 1 292 19178 2

Acknowledgements
The publisher would like to thank the following for their kind permission to reproduce their photographs:

(Key: b-bottom; c-centre; l-left; r-right; t-top)

Adam Gent: 77, 78t, 81b; **Alamy Stock Photo:** Mediscan 65br, 191, Momentum Creative Group 65bc; **Fotolia.com:** Pam 174r, sudok1 162t; **Pearson Education Ltd:** Josh Horwood, Studio8; 14, 19, 22tl, 22tr, 22bl, 22bc, 22br, 23tl, 23tc, 23tr, 23c, 23cr, 23bl, 23br, 25, 33t, 33b, 80, 80t, 86t, 90t, 92tl, 94, 95t, 95b, 96, 98, 101, 110l, 110c, 110r, 113tl, 113tr, 113bl, 113br, 121c, 122, 125t, 125c, 125b, 126t, 126c, 126cl, 126cr, 126bl, 126bc, 126br, 127tl, 127tc, 127tr, 127c, 127cl, 127cr, 127bl, 127br, 128tl, 128tr, 128bl, 128br, 130, 133tl, 133tc, 133tr, 136 (a), 136 (b), 136 (c), 136 (d), 136 (e), 136 (f), 137 (a), 137 (b), 137 (c), 137 (d), 137 (e), 137 (f), 137 (g), 137cr, 138 (a), 138 (b), 138 (c), 138 (d), 138 (e), 138 (f), 138 (g), 138 (h), 139t, 139b, 140tl, 140tr, 140cl, 140cr, 140b, 144, 147b, 150l, 150c, 150r, 151 (a), 151 (b), 151 (c), 151 (d), 151 (e), 151 (g), 152l, 152r, 153t, 153b, 154, 162b, 164l, 164r, 176c, 176r, 182t, 182c, 182b, 187, 199, 206, 207t, 207b, 209, 211, 214, 151f, 1, 23cl, 35, 43l, 43r, 45l, 45r, 47t, 47c, 47bl, 47br, 49, 50t, 50b, 51, 52tl, 52tr, 52bl, 52br, 54bl, 54br, 55t, 55b, 56, 59t, 59b, 62t, 62bl, 62br, 64l, 64r, 64bl, 64br, 72l, 72r, 73tl, 73tr, 73c, 73b, 74l, 74c, 74r, 75, 78b, 79, 80b, 81t, 86c, 86b, 87t, 87b, 88t, 88c, 88b, 89t, 89b, 90c, 90b, 91t, 91b, 92tr, 92bl, 93tl, 93tr, 93bl, 93br, 129l, 129r, 147t, 176l, David Sanderson 150t; **Shutterstock.com:** Christine Langer-Pueschel 186, Gang Liu 169, Johanna Goodyear 65bl, Pan Xunbin 174l, Peter ElvidgE 155, Piotr Krzeslak 65tr, Piotr Marcinski 121tl, 121tr, Rob Byron 174c, wellphoto 8

All other images © Pearson Education

The publisher would like to thank the following organisations for their kind permissions to reproduce their materials:

p.11 Figure 1.2 Gibbs' reflective cycle is used with permission of Oxford Brookes University; **p.17** Figure 1.3 The NARU triage sieve is reproduced by permission of the National Ambulance Resilience Unit (NARU); **p.25** Figure 1.4 Hand-washing technique is reproduced by permission of the World Health Organisation; **p.71** Figure 2.11 'Chain of Survival, Adult basic life support and automated external defibrillation', Resuscitation Council (UK). Reproduced with the kind permission of the Resuscitation Council (UK), https://www.resus.org.uk/resuscitation-guidelines/adult-basic-life-support-and-automated-external-defibrillation/#chain

The authors and publisher would like to thank the following:

The Faculty of Pre-Hospital Care, RCSEd, for reviewing and approving the content

Staffordshire Search and Rescue Team for their assistance in the production of the photographs (www.staffordshirelowlandrescue.org).

Models: Richard Archer, Sue Archer, Amy Bloor, Nigel Bowler, Sam Burt, Ned Coomes, Finlay Diamond, Edward Eldershaw, Evelyn Eldershaw, James Eldershaw, Rachel Eldershaw, Andy Faulkner, Susannah Fountain, Adam Gent, Penelope Gresford, Claire Gunn, Nic Gunn, Desmond Loo, Edward Malpass, Helen Morning, Robert Owen, Will Roberts, Lyndsay Sage, Leanne Savigar
Reviewers: John Amos (SBStJ, CERT HE, MCPara), Nigel Hinson and Neil Proven

Claire Gunn and Lyndsay Sage for their continuous, unwavering support of Nic Gunn and Adam Gent. Susannah Fountain for her professionalism, diligence and dedication towards the production of this book.

Websites
Pearson Education Limited is not responsible for the content of any external internet sites. It is essential for tutors to preview each website before using it in class so as to ensure that the URL is still accurate, relevant and appropriate. We suggest that tutors bookmark useful websites and consider enabling students to access them through the school/college intranet.

Note from the publisher
Pearson has robust editorial processes, including answer and fact checks, to ensure the accuracy of the content in this publication, and every effort is made to ensure this publication is free of errors. We are, however, only human, and occasionally errors do occur. Pearson is not liable for any misunderstandings that arise as a result of errors in this publication, but it is our priority to ensure that the content is accurate. If you spot an error, please do contact us at resourcescorrections@pearson.com so we can make sure it is corrected.

Contents

How to use this book

Welcome to First Person on Scene (Second edition), for your Pearson BTEC Level 4 Certificate and Extended Certificate professional qualifications.

The Faculty of Pre-Hospital Care of the Royal College of Surgeons of Edinburgh created this qualification initially with IHCD (then part of Edexcel – now Pearson). They worked with Pearson in developing the new qualification and in reviewing the current handbook.

The book has been written by pre-hospital care professionals to equip first responders to support the emergency services in the evaluation and management of casualties. As a first responder, your role is to respond to, and manage, both medical and trauma emergencies from the point of arrival, to the handover to the next echelon of care. You will study a range of units which will help you to gain an understanding of the roles and responsibilities involved, together with the skills and knowledge required to provide emergency care and manage trauma situations and medical conditions.

The qualification is for learners who work in, or who want to work in, the pre-hospital care industry as first responders. In some cases you may be acting as a first responder as part of a secondary role in an industry which requires first responders to have a greater breadth of knowledge and skill than is provided by first-aid qualifications.

The qualification gives you the opportunity to develop knowledge related to the pre-hospital care industry. This includes how your role fits into the wider sector, as well as the responsibilities of the first responder, established practices relating to the safeguarding of children and vulnerable adults, and the prevention and control of infection.

How your BTEC is structured

The book is divided into five units, the first of which is externally assessed by means of an online assessment. The remaining four units are assessed internally with assessments devised by centres running the course. Unit 5 is a synoptic unit designed to help you explore and use the knowledge and understanding gained in the first four units to manage incidents competently in simulated environments.

The content aligns with the Certificate and the Extended Certificate specifications and is structured such that you can identify content which is applicable to the Extended Certificate only.

Features of this book

There are a number of different features in the book to support your learning.

▶ Key terms to help explain unfamiliar terminology.
▶ Cross-referencing across the content.
▶ Quick checks to ensure you understand the learning outcomes.
▶ Tips which provide additional, useful, information.
▶ Step-by-step guidance on what to do in a medical emergency.
▶ Assessment activities to help you prepare for end-of-unit assessment.
▶ Further reading for wider research into some of the topics covered.

Features that explain what your learning is about

Getting to know your unit

This section introduces the unit and explains how you will be assessed. It gives an overview of what will be covered and will help you to understand **why** you are doing the things you are asked to do in the unit. The Learning outcomes and Assessment criteria are provided in separate tables for both the Certificate and Extended Certificate specifications, for each unit, so that you can see at a glance what you are required to do.

Getting started

This appears at the start of every unit and is designed to get you thinking about the unit and what it involves. This feature will also help you to identify what you may already know about some of the topics in the unit and acts as a starting point for understanding the skills and knowledge you will need to develop to complete the unit.

Features that help you to build your knowledge

Key terms

Concise and simple definitions are provided for key words, phrases and concepts, allowing you to have, at a glance, a clear understanding of the key ideas in each unit.

Link

This shows any links between units or within the same unit, helping you to identify where the knowledge you have learned elsewhere will help you to achieve the requirements of the unit. Remember that, although the book is made up of five units, there are common themes that are explored from different perspectives across the whole of your course.

Quick check

These are questions that appear at points throughout the unit to help you recap on what you have learned.

Quick tip

Practical hints and tips for techniques are provided to give guidance when using equipment or carrying out procedures.

Step by step:

This practical feature gives step-by-step descriptions of particular processes or tasks in the unit, occasionally including a photo or artwork for each step, or certain steps. This will help you to understand the key stages in the process and help you to carry out the process yourself.

Further reading and resources

This contains a list of other resources – such as books, journals, articles or websites – you can use to expand your knowledge of the unit content. This is a good opportunity for you to take responsibility for your own learning, as well as preparing you for research tasks you may need to do academically or professionally.

Features connected to your assessment

All the units in your course are mandatory and these are either:
- externally assessed or
- internally assessed.

This course has one externally assessed unit (Unit 1). The features that support you in preparing for assessment are below. But first, what is the difference between these two different types of units?

Externally assessed units

Unit 1 gives you the opportunity to present what you have learned in the unit in a different way. For this unit, you will complete an online assessment consisting of multiple-choice questions, set directly by Pearson, in controlled conditions.

Internally assessed units

Units 2–5 will be internally assessed. This involves you completing a series of assignments, set and marked by your centre. The assignments you complete could allow you to demonstrate your learning in a number of different ways, from a written report, to a presentation, to a video recording and observation statements of you completing a practical task. Whatever the method, you will need to make sure you have clear evidence of what you have achieved and how you completed it.

Assessment practice (C, EC) 3.1, 3.2

These features give you the opportunity to practise some of the skills you will need when you are assessed on your unit. Coverage of the Assessment criteria is shown in the top right hand corner of this box: (C) indicates coverage of the Certificate specification, and (EC) indicates coverage of the Extended Certificate. They do not fully reflect the actual assessment tasks, but will help you prepare for them.

Plan – Do – Review
You'll also find handy advice on how to plan, complete and evaluate your work after you have completed it. This is designed to get you thinking about the best way to complete your work and to build your skills and experience before doing the actual assessment. These prompt questions are designed to help you think about how and why you do things.

About the Authors

Adam Gent

Adam has been involved with the development and delivery of first aid and pre-hospital training since 2000, specialising in delivering care in remote environments. Originally an outdoor instructor and geography teacher, he has worked across most of the mountainous regions of Europe, as well as Tanzania, Dominican Republic, Goa, Borneo, Dubai, Ukraine and Tajikistan. Adam is a Fellow of the Royal Geographical Society, Senior Associate of the Royal Society of Medicine and Member of the Royal College of Surgeons of Edinburgh Faculty of Pre-Hospital Care. Adam was a co-author for the First Person on Scene Level 4 qualification specification for Pearson.

Nic Gunn

Nic is an HCPC-registered paramedic (Health and Care Professions Council), a qualified teacher and a member of Staffordshire Search and Rescue Team. Having gained his PGCE from Keele University, he became a secondary school teacher while also volunteering as a community first responder. Nic began his training career while working in the leisure industry delivering first aid and National Pool Lifeguard training. He left teaching and completed a Foundation Degree in Paramedic Science and now works as a paramedic for an NHS trust. He was a co-author for the First Person on Scene Level 4 qualification specification for Pearson.

About the Faculty of Pre-Hospital Care of the Royal College of Surgeons of Edinburgh

The Faculty of Pre-Hospital Care of the Royal College of Surgeons of Edinburgh has very much embraced the continued development and reach of clinical care delivered at all levels in all areas of the pre-hospital environment. It works to support, promote and educate care providers from the non-professional medic to the highest specialised clinician, collaborating with multiple agencies to achieve this.

The Faculty of Pre-Hospital Care of the Royal College of Surgeons of Edinburgh has reviewed and approved the content.

Guidelines

Please note that the guidelines below have been followed during the writing of this book.

The Royal College of Surgeons of Edinburgh, Faculty of Pre-Hospital Care – consensus statements.

UK Ambulance Service Clinical Practice Guidelines (JRCALC) 2016.

The Resuscitation Council (UK) Guidelines 2015.

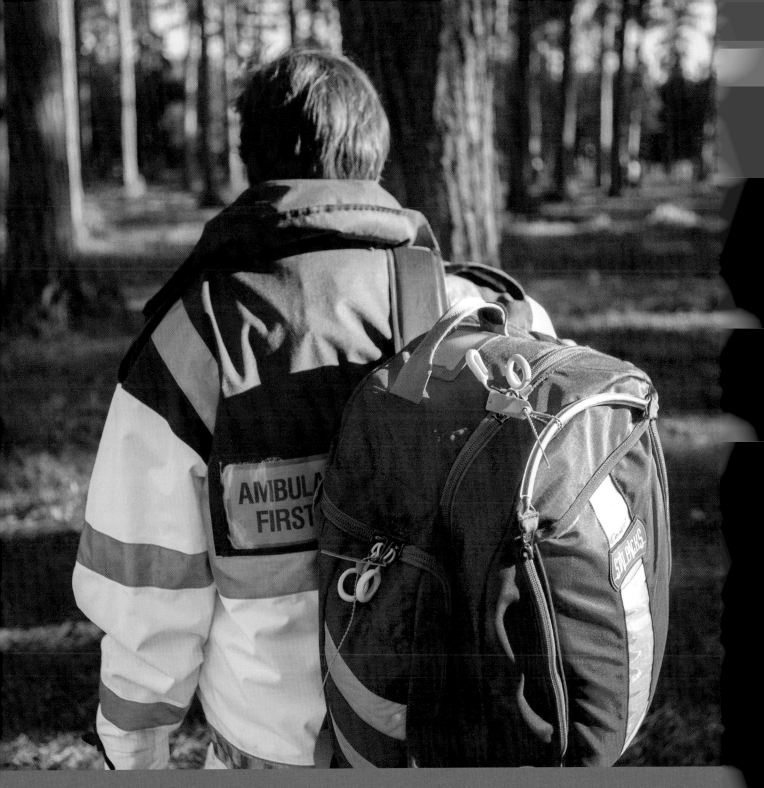

Understanding the Roles and Responsibilities of the First Responder

1

Getting to know your unit

Providing care in an emergency requires a wide range of knowledge that underpins the practical aspect of emergency care. Ensuring you have a sound understanding of this knowledge will help you to make confident and competent decisions about what actions to take in the event of a medical emergency so that you can manage an incident effectively from the point of your arrival at the scene to handing over to definitive pre-hospital care providers.

In this unit you will learn about the responsibilities you have when carrying out emergency care. You will learn about how to manage the scene and those in attendance at the incident to keep yourself, bystanders and casualties safe from a variety of potential hazards and risks. You will gain an understanding of how to safeguard the vulnerable people you may meet and the actions you should take should you become aware of a potential safeguarding concern. You will go on to learn how to prevent and control infection, including the responsibilities of both yourself and your employer. Finally, you will explore the processes and procedures that the first responder is responsible for following the management of the casualty.

While this unit assesses your underpinning knowledge and understanding, you will also have the opportunity to explore the practical skills that apply to these roles and responsibilities. In doing so, you will begin to develop the associated skills required to confidently and competently manage incidents involving a range of casualties requiring emergency care as presented in *Unit 5: Developing the Competencies of Incident Management for the First Responder.*

How you will be assessed

This Level 3 unit will be externally assessed with an on-screen multiple-choice test. The test will have 23 questions and will use a variety of question types, such as:

▶ selecting one answer from four options

▶ selecting two answers from five options

▶ dragging and dropping answers into the correct place

▶ line-matching items to the correct options.

This is a pass-or-fail exam and there is no opportunity to gain different grades dependant upon your score.

This unit comprises six learning outcomes. Each learning objective has a number of assessment criteria shown in the following table. It is this assessment criteria against which your knowledge will be tested during the examination.

Each assessment criteria has some 'command words' associated with it – see Table 1.1 for a list of what these command words are asking you to do.

Command words used in this unit

▶ **Table 1.1**

Command word	Definition – what it is asking you to do
Identify	State the key fact(s) about a topic or subject.
Describe	Give a full account of all the information about a topic, including all the relevant details of any features.
Explain	Make an idea, situation or problem clear to your reader by describing it in detail, including any relevant data or facts.
Use	Apply your knowledge in order to use a piece of equipment effectively.

Unit 1 Learning outcomes and Assessment criteria (Certificate)

▶ **Table 1.2**

Learning outcome 1: Understand the first responder's responsibilities

Assessment criteria	
1.1	Explain the primary responsibilities of the first responder
1.2	Explain how the first responder can maintain their knowledge and skills over time
1.3	Describe how the first responder can protect themselves from false allegations

Learning outcome 2: Understand the safe management of the scene

Assessment criteria	
2.1	Describe the capabilities of emergency service responders
2.2	Explain the principles of scene management
2.3	Use the triage sieve to effectively prioritise the management of multiple casualties

Learning outcome 3: Understand how to manage own and others' safety when attending incidents as the first responder

Assessment criteria	
3.1	Identify hazards that pose a risk to the safety of self and others when attending incidents
3.2	Identify the priority in which the first responder should ensure the safety of those present at the incident
3.3	Explain the correct selection of Personal Protective Equipment (PPE) to be worn to maintain own and others' safety when attending incidents
3.4	Describe strategies that can be employed to reduce potential risks to the first responder

Learning outcome 4: Understand the principles relating to infection prevention and control

Assessment criteria	
4.1	Describe the responsibilities of the first responder in relation to infection prevention and control
4.2	Describe how to maintain professional standards of personal hygiene
4.3	Describe the principles of hand hygiene
4.4	Describe the chain of infection

Learning outcome 5: Understand the safeguarding of children and vulnerable adults

Assessment criteria	
5.1	Identify signs of potential abuse
5.2	Describe the actions to be taken if a safeguarding issue is suspected
5.3	Describe the actions the first responder should take if a safeguarding issue is disclosed

Learning outcome 6: Understand post-incident procedures and vulnerable adults

Assessment criteria	
6.1	Explain the principles of an effective clinical handover
6.2	Describe the components of a Patient Report Form
6.3	Describe the steps to be taken to ensure equipment is serviceable and available post-incident
6.4	Explain when the first responder should seek help with their own mental wellbeing

Unit 1 Learning outcomes and Assessment criteria (Extended Certificate)

▶ **Table 1.3**

Learning outcome 1: Understand the first responder's responsibilities

Assessment criteria	
1.1	Explain the primary responsibilities of the first responder
1.2	Explain how the first responder can maintain their knowledge and skills over time
1.3	Describe how the first responder can protect themselves from false allegations

Learning outcome 2: Understand the safe management of the scene

Assessment criteria	
2.1	Describe the capabilities of emergency service responders
2.2	Explain the principles of scene management
2.3	Use the triage sieve to effectively prioritise the management of multiple casualties

Learning outcome 3: Understand how to manage own and others' safety when attending incidents as the first responder

Assessment criteria	
3.1	Identify hazards that pose a risk to the safety of self and others when attending incidents
3.2	Identify the priority in which the first responder should ensure the safety of those present at the incident
3.3	Explain the correct selection of Personal Protective Equipment (PPE) to be worn to maintain own and others' safety when attending incidents
3.4	Describe strategies that can be employed to reduce potential risks to the first responder

Learning outcome 4: Understand the principles relating to infection prevention and control

Assessment criteria	
4.1	Describe the responsibilities of the first responder in relation to infection prevention and control
4.2	Describe how to maintain professional standards of personal hygiene
4.3	Describe the principles of hand hygiene
4.4	Describe the chain of infection

Learning outcome 5: Understand the safeguarding of children and vulnerable adults

Assessment criteria	
5.1	Identify signs of potential abuse
5.2	Describe the actions to be taken if a safeguarding issue is suspected
5.3	Describe the actions the first responder should take if a safeguarding issue is disclosed

Learning outcome 6: Understand post-incident procedures

Assessment criteria	
6.1	Explain the principles of an effective clinical handover
6.2	Describe the components of a Patient Report Form
6.3	Describe the steps to be taken to ensure equipment is serviceable and available post-incident
6.4	Explain when the first responder should seek help with their own mental wellbeing

Getting started

Think about what might be involved in the first responder's role. What personal qualities do you have that will enable you to become an effective first responder?

Understand the first responder's responsibilities

The role of the first responder is a complex one. At the scene of an emergency you have many different responsibilities and you have to be able to move between these depending upon the scene you are presented with. The scene of an emergency can be dynamic and challenging for you and for the people involved.

Safety

Your first and most important role at the scene of an emergency is safety. You must prioritise safety in the following order:

1 **Your safety.** The most important person at the scene is you, and you must recognise when it is safe to approach a situation and when it is not. If the scene is unsafe and you become a casualty yourself, you will be unable to help anyone else.

2 **People at the scene.** You must then consider the safety of other people at the scene: these may be bystanders, people administering first aid or other emergency services personnel. If you are able to spot a hazard that they may not be aware of, you must give clear instructions to keep them safe.

3 **The casualty.** Only when you have ensured your safety and that of others at the scene, can you consider the safety of the casualty. Do you need to move the casualty immediately to keep them safe?

Recognising when a scene is unsafe and taking simple steps to rectify the situation is very important (see **Figure 1.1**).

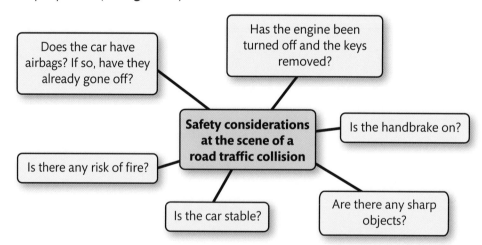

Figure 1.1 What must you consider at the scene of a road traffic collision?

If you can make the scene a safe place to be for everyone, then do so. If the scene is unsafe for you (for example, if the car airbags have not yet deployed and you need to get into the car to assess the casualty), then you must move away and summon assistance from the appropriate agencies.

Step 1-2-3

The Step 1-2-3 procedure provides safety triggers for first responders and other emergency personnel. It refers to the number of casualties (one, two, or three or more) at a scene. Use it if you have multiple casualties and cannot immediately identify the cause of the incident as you approach it. In these cases, you need to give special consideration to your own safety.

For example, if you arrive at the scene of a road traffic collision where there are three casualties, the cause of their injuries is obvious and you can easily identify the other hazards to your own safety, then it may be safe to approach. However, if you arrive at a scene where there are two or more casualties suffering from illness or injury, and the cause is not apparent, you should question why this might be, to avoid becoming a casualty yourself. There are many reasons why there may be more than one ill or injured casualty in the same place, such as:

▶ chemical release

▶ terrorism

▶ other hazardous materials.

Imagine you have arrived at a shopping centre to find one casualty lying unconscious on the floor. Ask yourself: Is the situation suspicious? Are there additional casualties? If there is just one casualty, you should approach them following your normal procedures and protocols. However, if there are two casualties, approach the scene with caution for your own safety. If there are three casualties and no obvious cause, do not approach them; summon assistance from the emergency services and give them as detailed a description as you can of the situation.

As a guide, follow these rules:

Step 1	One casualty	Approach normally
Step 2	Two casualties	Approach with caution
Step 3	Three or more casualties (including any other responders)	Do not approach; request assistance

Summoning assistance

Even though you may be the first person on scene at an incident, this does not mean you are expected to deal with the situation on your own. It is important that you summon assistance as quickly as possible. Who, where and what that assistance will be will vary depending on the situation but you need to know who can come to your aid in your operational environment. Some examples could be:

▶ other team members

▶ other people at the scene

▶ Police

▶ Fire and Rescue Service

▶ Ambulance Service

▶ Mountain Rescue

▶ Coastguard

▶ RNLI Lifeboats

▶ Lowland Rescue.

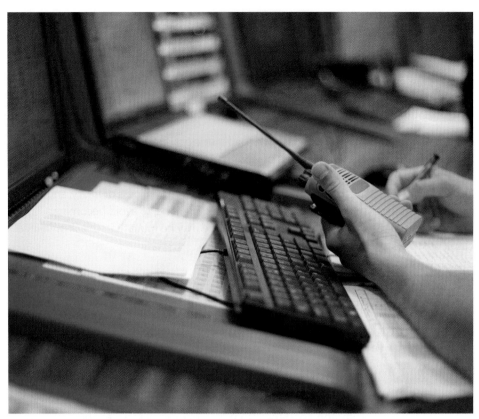

Which agencies can come to your aid in an operational environment?

Providing initial management and taking control

As the first person on scene, it is likely that you will be the most medically qualified person at an incident until assistance arrives. It is key to your role that you are able to manage the casualty effectively until help that is more qualified arrives.

Other people at the scene, and the casualty, will start to look to you to take control as you arrive. Stay calm. This helps to instil confidence in your ability and will help you when you want other people at the scene to do something to help.

Casualty assessment

A significant part of the role of the first person on scene is to perform a methodical and thorough casualty assessment. There are many parts to this assessment, including physical examination and **history taking**, and this is where you will spend a large proportion of time while undertaking your duties. Without this you will be unable to manage the casualty effectively.

Managing casualties within your scope of practice

When you are managing a casualty, it is important to know what management skills you have available. It is also important that you do not deviate from your scope of practice. Your scope of practice is defined by what you have been taught to do proficiently and what your organisation allows you to do. Performing interventions outside this scope of practice could have legal consequences for you and harmful implications for the casualty.

Key term

History taking – asking questions about what has happened, finding out what signs and symptoms the casualty has, asking about the casualty's past medical history and current medications.

Link

The process of casualty assessment is explored in further detail in Unit 2 on page 42.

Casualty reporting

You must provide an accurate record of events on a **Patient Report Form (PRF)**. A PRF becomes part of the casualty's medical story from their initial management from you through to **definitive care** at hospital. Where possible, it should be completed and given to the next **echelon of care** when you hand over the casualty. There are times when this is not possible as the casualty is critically ill and you have been managing them. In this situation, complete the report form as soon as possible, for example while the ambulance crew are loading the casualty onto the ambulance. If you have not been able to complete the report form before the casualty leaves the scene, you need to ensure you follow your local policies and procedures with regard to what you do with the completed paperwork.

Providing interim management of incidents while awaiting the next level of care

While it is important to take control of the scene and provide initial management of the casualty it is just as important to be able to hand over responsibility for some tasks when other emergency services arrive. For example, when you are dealing with a road traffic collision and the police arrive, you can hand over any traffic management for safety to them and you can hand over responsibility for the casualty's management to the ambulance service. It may, however, be that you are required to continue to help and support the next level of care, with further tasks under their guidance and instruction after you have handed over the responsibility.

Knowledge and skills

After you have successfully completed your course you must ensure that you keep the knowledge and skills you have gained at the required standard, recognising your own skill decay and identifying methods of maintaining your knowledge (see following). Recording and tracking your own practice will help you identify skills that you have not recently used and will enable you to recognise any skill decay. You could keep a log (electronically or manually) of each skill you have performed to identify when there is a need to revisit each skill before skill decay occurs and you are unable to manage a casualty effectively.

Understanding the importance of being physically and mentally fit to perform the role

Interacting with people when they are in pain or under stress can be both a mentally and physically demanding job. It is important that you take time to look after yourself. Some elements of your own health you will need to consider are:

▶ sleep
▶ nutrition
▶ hydration
▶ physical fitness
▶ immunisations
▶ occupational health screening
▶ having sufficient rest time in between shifts and throughout the week.

Link

See page 32 for an example of a completed PRF.

Key terms

Patient Report Form (PRF) – this is a legal and confidential record about a casualty, including details such as incident date/time/location, casualty information, responder's details and physical assessment.

Definitive care – a place where the casualty is able to have all of the treatment that they require, e.g. hospital.

Echelon of care – the next level of care, which can provide more qualified help for the casualty, e.g. the ambulance service.

Quick check

Can you identify the roles and responsibilities of the first responder? Can you expand on this by writing a short sentence to describe each one?

Maintenance of knowledge and skills

Taking responsibility for your own learning

You need to make sure that you:

▶ communicate any training needs to your supervisor/mentor/responsible officer

▶ record and track your own practice to help you identify skills that you have not recently used to make sure you can identify any skills decay

▶ review your own practice and performance after an incident. It is important to look at both the positives and the negatives, and at what you can learn from every incident.

Methods of maintaining your knowledge and skills

There are different ways that you can keep yourself up to date with the latest practices and maintain your knowledge and skills at the expected level. Choose the correct method for different skills, e.g. if you have not completed a life support incident for some time, it may be beneficial to practise this as a practical skill on a manikin, whereas if you need to refresh your knowledge on signs and symptoms of a heart attack, some self-directed study may be more appropriate. Only you know how you learn most effectively, so choose a method that works for you. Some examples of these methods are:

▶ ongoing professional practice – attending as many incidents as you can; the more often you complete a task, the better you remember it

▶ attending seminars and conferences

▶ undertaking self-directed study, such as reading this book, plus relevant articles in journals or academic publications

▶ practical skill training

▶ mentoring

▶ work placement

▶ undertaking further formal training or study

▶ reflective practice – look back at what you have done and think about how it went (how you felt, what went well, what didn't go well and what you could do differently next time).

Quick check

Look at the following **Figure 1.2** showing Gibbs' reflective cycle. Using this cycle, think about an incident (either real or hypothetical) and write a paragraph about what happened at each stage of the cycle. What action plan could you use if the same incident were to happen again?

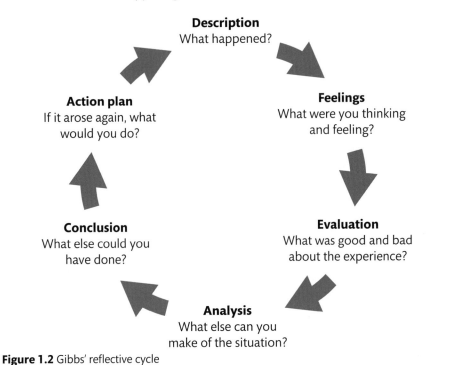

Figure 1.2 Gibbs' reflective cycle

Protecting yourself from allegations

Consent

For you to be able to perform an assessment or to manage a casualty's condition you need to have their agreement for this to happen. This is called 'consent'. A casualty can refuse assessment and management where they have capacity to do so. In cases where the casualty is unconscious you do not need to gain consent to assess and manage them as this would be impractical. For consent to be valid it must be given by the casualty voluntarily and they should have all the facts to be able to make an informed decision. Ask the casualty if you can assess them at the beginning of your interactions with them.

The casualty must also have capacity to make that decision, which means they must be able to retain the information you are telling them, be able to use that information to weigh up the options and be able to communicate their decision to you. There are times when a casualty's capacity may be impaired, such as:

▶ mental health conditions

▶ **dementia**

▶ severe learning difficulties

▶ intoxication

▶ brain injury.

Key term

Dementia – an umbrella term used to describe a range of disorders (e.g. Alzheimer's disease) that can affect the casualty's brain function. There are many types, and symptoms can include memory and communication problems.

The decision whether a casualty has capacity is one that is normally completed by an appropriately trained healthcare professional. It is a decision that is not taken lightly. Where you are presented with a casualty who is refusing treatment but who you believe may lack capacity, it is important to seek assistance as soon as possible so the assessment can take place promptly. As a first responder, you will not be expected to make the decision as to whether a casualty has capacity or not, and you should follow your local policy and guidelines.

All of your decisions with regard to consent should be clearly documented on the PRF, explaining that consent was either given or refused. Where a casualty has consented to some assessments or managements but not others, you should clearly document this.

Being alone with a casualty

Sometimes, being alone with a casualty is unavoidable, but wherever you are dealing with a vulnerable casualty it is important to try to have a witness. This could be a friend or relative of the casualty, a colleague or a member of the emergency services. You need to be able to justify your actions.

Accurate and extensive recording

Accurate and extensive recording of each incident on the PRF provides evidence that can be used to justify your actions. This should include any examinations you performed. You should be able to show why a particular examination was necessary. For example, if a casualty has been kicked by a horse in the chest, it would be necessary to expose the casualty's chest (in as discreet a way as possible) to be able to complete an examination. You should report this on the PRF.

Assessment practice 1.1   (C, EC) 1.1, 1.2, 1.3

Susannah is starting her First Person on Scene training next month and has emailed you asking for advice on what the job involves. She has sent the following questions:

1 What is the role of the first responder?

2 How do I keep up to date with latest practices?

3 How can I help protect myself in case I am accused of anything?

Plan
- Does Susannah have any prior knowledge about a first responder's role?
- What do I need to tell her to answer each of her three points?
- How can I structure my answer most effectively?

Do
- If Susannah has no prior knowledge, I need to explain terminology and procedures clearly.

Review
- Have I included enough detail to help her get ready for the course?

Understand the safe management of the scene

Emergency services

It is important to be able to summon assistance from other responders at the scene of an incident to assist you in managing the casualties. To be able to do this effectively you must be aware of the different roles each responder performs. This is also useful when you arrive at a scene where other responders are already working. There is a need to work together and to communicate to ensure the scene remains safe and the casualty receives the correct care. Other responders you may have a need to call upon are:

▶ Police

▶ Fire and Rescue Service

▶ Ambulance Service

▶ Mountain Rescue

▶ Coastguard

▶ RNLI Lifeboats

▶ Lowland Rescue.

It is important to understand which of these services are available in your operational area and their individual capabilities. These capabilities can vary from area to area but you need to be aware of the general abilities of each type of responder.

▶ **Table 1.4**

Responder	Capabilities
Police	▶ Managing health and safety at the scene ▶ Traffic management, e.g. closing roads ▶ Evidence preservation ▶ Criminal investigation ▶ Providing assistance with aggressive or potentially violent people
Fire and Rescue Service	▶ Firefighting ▶ Managing health and safety, e.g. stabilising a car at the scene of a road traffic collision (RTC) ▶ Extrication, e.g. providing better access to a casualty at the scene of an RTC or industrial accident by using cutting equipment ▶ Providing access and rescue of a casualty, e.g. rope rescue, working at heights ▶ Rescue of a casualty in a hazardous environment
Ambulance Service	▶ Casualty assessment ▶ Treatment ▶ Transportation of the casualty to definitive care ▶ All ambulance services have access to a Hazardous Area Response Team – teams of paramedics who have special training in accessing and treating casualties in difficult environments
Mountain Rescue	▶ Mountain extrication ▶ Providing rope access to a casualty ▶ Search and rescue ▶ Water rescue
Coastguard	▶ Managing health and safety ▶ Providing access to a casualty ▶ Extrication of a casualty ▶ Search and Rescue, including provision of Search and Rescue helicopters
RNLI Lifeboats	▶ Lifeboat provision at sea and some inland water areas ▶ Search and rescue in the water
Lowland Rescue	▶ Search and rescue ▶ Water rescue ▶ Lowland extrication

Link

See page 6 for more information on safety priorities.

Scene management

In addition to the safety priorities mentioned earlier in the unit, there are many other aspects to consider when managing a scene.

As you arrive at a scene, it is important to perform a scene survey. This must include:

▶ safety

▶ establishing the cause

▶ environment

▶ triage

▶ additional resources.

Establishing the cause

Key term

Mechanism of injury – the method through which damage to skin, muscles, organs and bones occurs. This will help determine the seriousness of the injury.

When first arriving at the scene of an incident it is important to attempt to establish the cause. This is particularly important in situations in which casualties have traumatic injuries. This is called the **mechanism of injury**. By understanding the mechanism of injury you can predict the potential areas and extent of the injuries the casualty may have suffered. Do this when you arrive at the incident. Ask yourself questions to try to work out what has happened.

For example, you are called to a child casualty who is lying on the ground in a playground.

▶ Has the child fallen off a climbing frame? If so, how high was it?

▶ Did they land on concrete, sand, tarmac or grass?

▶ What position are they lying in?

Asking yourself questions will help you to predict traumatic injuries such as a spinal cord injury.

Impact of the environment on the management of the scene

There are external factors that can affect the management of a casualty. These factors can influence your decisions about the additional resources you may require to successfully manage the scene. They can be categorised in the following four ways.

Weather conditions

The weather may influence the time it takes for you and any additional resources to reach the casualty. If it is snowing and the roads are difficult to navigate, is there anything you can do to manage the scene in the meantime? Conversely, on a warm day, do you need to create some shade for the casualty, or move them safely to a shady area?

Access to the scene

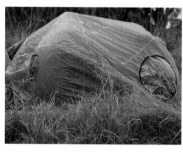

An emergency shelter

There are many situations in which access to the casualty may be difficult. You may need to consider summoning assistance. For example:

▶ at height

▶ underground

▶ on steep ground.

You must remember to ensure your safety first then consider the order or priority of events to ensure the safety of others.

 Self → **Other people at the scene** → **Casualty**

You may not be able to gain access to a casualty's property if they have fallen and they are unable to reach the door to unlock it. In this case the police would be required to force entry to allow you to assess the casualty.

Egress from the scene

Egress occurs when responders and casualties are able to leave the scene safely. You must think about how you will extract the casualty from the scene and how you can help them reach definitive care. Where egress is not straightforward, liaise with other agencies to formulate a plan to ensure the safety of all the responders and casualties. This may include specialist stretchers or helicopters.

Complicated egress of a casualty can be something as simple as removing the casualty on a stretcher when they are located in an upstairs room. If you combine this with factors such as the size and weight of a casualty, a bend in the steep staircase and a narrow hallway, this can quickly become problematic.

Location of the casualty

Access and egress might be issues in remote environments such as mountains, country parks or woodland. Consider whether specialist services are available in these situations; for example, the local mountain rescue team or forest rangers.

Working in urban environments also presents challenges. For example:

▸ Being on, or near, roads can be dangerous. Consider requesting the closure of a road for your own safety and that of the casualty. Road noise can also be a problem when communicating with the casualty and others.

▸ Construction sites and factories can have dangerous equipment and noise issues.

▸ Being on, or near, water can be dangerous.

Number of casualties and severity of injury

When there are more casualties than there are first responders, you must start the process of **triage** to decide which casualty you are going to assess and manage first. You should use this information to update other responders and to summon assistance. You must assess and manage the casualties that are most ill or injured and perform a rapid assessment of their injuries. You must prioritise by deciding which is the most life-threatening condition. Consider the following order when deciding which casualties to assess first:

1 any casualty with a catastrophic bleed
2 any casualty with an **occluded airway**
3 any casualty who is not breathing
4 any casualty who is unconscious but breathing
5 any casualty with signs of abnormal breathing
6 any casualty with signs of abnormal circulation
7 any remaining injuries based on the severity.

Key terms

Triage – deciding the order of treatment when faced with multiple casualties or multiple injuries.

Occluded airway – a blocked airway where no air can pass to and from the lungs.

Link

For more information on catastrophic haemorrhage, see Unit 2, page 45.

Link

For more information on casualties who are not breathing, see Unit 2, page 72, Agonal breathing.

Link

In Unit 2, you will learn how to assess a casualty and the principles used to prioritise them.

Quick check

After assessing scene safety, what is the next step you should take when managing a scene?

You may be presented with two casualties, one who is shouting for help and the other who is quiet. Although the vocal casualty may be distracting, it is important to assess the quiet casualty first as they may be experiencing an illness or injury that is preventing them from asking for help. The shouting casualty is clearly breathing without difficulty and, as such, does not require your immediate attention.

Additional resources

Once you have all of this information, you can request the appropriate support from other services. It may be that you have radio contact with ambulance control and can request further resources. You should follow your local policy and procedures.

Major incident reporting

Where an incident may have an impact on an emergency service's ability to perform its normal duties, they may declare a major incident. All emergency services follow the principles set out by the Joint Emergency Services Interoperability Programme (JESIP). This was formed in 2012 to address recommendations made following reports on major incidents. In order to create a shared situational awareness of an incident for all responding services across all agencies, a METHANE report is passed to their control.

The stages of a METHANE report are:

▸ **M**ajor incident declared or standby

▸ **E**xact location

▸ **T**ype of incident, e.g. a collapsed building

▸ **H**azards

▸ **A**ccess and egress

▸ **N**umber, type and severity of casualties

▸ **E**mergency services on scene and summoned.

It is important that this information is passed on at the earliest opportunity to allow all agencies to share the information and to ensure they can send the correct response. This METHANE report can, and should, be updated as a situation changes.

Major incident triage

Where there are significant casualties at a major incident, casualties must be triaged using the following tool – a triage sieve – which shows the order in which casualties should be treated (see **Figure 1.3**).

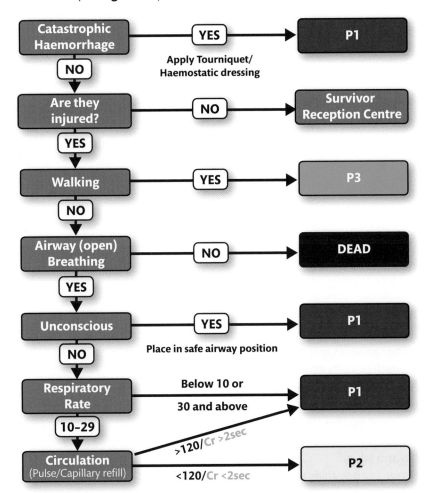

Figure 1.3 The NARU (National Ambulance Resilience Unit) triage sieve

Once triage has taken place, casualties are moved to the appropriate location where treatment can begin. Casualties are managed in the order of:

▶ P1 (Priority 1)

▶ P2 (Priority 2)

▶ P3 (Priority 3).

Casualties who are P1 or P2 will need to be moved by responders and P3 casualties will be sent to a marked location.

Pen is considering a career in the emergency services.

1 To help her decide which service will suit her, complete this table:

▶ **Table 1.5**

Responder	Capabilities
Police	
Fire and Rescue Service	
Ambulance Service	
Mountain Rescue	
Coastguard	
RNLI Lifeboats	
Lowland Rescue	

2 Having decided to join the ambulance service, and after completing her training, Pen arrives at the scene of a road traffic collision on a busy dual carriageway. Describe the steps she would take when assessing the scene.

3 Pen has decided that this is a major incident with 25 casualties. She is first on scene. What would be in her METHANE report?

4 Pen is then asked to complete triage of the casualties and is given the triage tool. In which category would each casualty be placed?

   a) Casualty lying on the floor with a lower leg injury. Unable to walk with a pulse of 130 and a respiration rate of 30.

   b) Casualty lying unconscious on the floor. Breathing normally.

   c) Casualty walking towards her, uninjured.

   d) Casualty walking towards her with an arm injury.

   e) Casualty lying unresponsive on the floor, not breathing with an open airway.

Plan

What information do I need to complete the task?

Where will I find that information?

Do

Use your imagination for questions 2 and 3. Think about a location near you and base your answers on that.

Review

Have I included everything I need to give as much detail as I can?

Understand how to manage own and others' safety when attending incidents as the first responder

Hazards

You must be able to identify hazards as you approach a scene. This will help to keep you and others safe. Some of the hazards are listed next.

▶ **The mental state of the casualty:** not every casualty wants your help and some may not think they need your help. They may be distressed, anxious or delusional. A casualty who has just been assaulted will need a different approach to an elderly casualty who has fallen. As a first responder, you need to be able to vary your approach according to the situation.

- **Drug and/or alcohol involvement:** both alcohol and drugs have a potential to change the behaviour of the casualty. Be mindful if you suspect that they may be under the influence of either. As you conduct your scene survey look around the area for any evidence, for example empty bottles or drug paraphernalia.

- **Falling objects:** there may be a risk of falling objects in some environments such as working at the bottom of a rock face. Manage the risk appropriately by wearing the correct Personal Protective Equipment (PPE) (see page 22) or by withdrawing and summoning assistance if necessary.

- **Fire:** you must not attempt to rescue a casualty from an active fire as this presents a significant risk to your own life. You should, instead, withdraw and summon assistance. You may, however, be asked to treat casualties following their rescue to a safe place. You also need to be aware of areas where there is a risk of fire. Remember that for a fire to take place, all three elements (shown in the Fire Triangle in Unit 2, **Figure 2.14**) must be in place: heat, oxygen and fuel. Consider this as you approach a scene.

- **Sharps:** as a first responder, you will have contact with sharp objects such as needles, broken glass or drug paraphernalia. The correct PPE should be worn to help protect yourself against infection and to prevent injury. You should be cautious when working in areas where sharp objects and needles are present.

- **Infection:** you are at risk of infection when assessing and managing a casualty. It is important that the correct equipment is used to help prevent this.

- **Utilities, i.e. gas, electricity:** utilities such as gas, electricity and water can pose risks to your safety if they are faulty. Household gas has a detectable smell. Where this is strong, you should withdraw from the premises, with the casualty if possible, and summon assistance from the fire service. You should also be aware of carbon monoxide poisoning and recognise the signs and symptoms.

- **Animals:** when a casualty calls for an ambulance, they will be asked to lock away any pets to enable you to carry out your assessment easily and safely. Not all animals will be found in the casualty's home, however. Cattle, horses and other livestock can cause significant harm when you are called to more remote locations. When dealing with casualties in the street who have dogs with them, it is important to think about how that dog will react when you are trying to help their owner who is unwell. Dogs can become very defensive and potentially dangerous. If their owner is unable to move to tether the dog, think about summoning assistance from the police dog handlers to secure the dog to allow you to assess the casualty.

- **Traffic:** this is not only a problem at a road traffic collision but can also be an issue when dealing with a casualty in the street. Is fast-moving traffic a hazard to your safety and that of the casualty? If you have arrived in a vehicle, think about where and how you can park it in accordance with your training and local policy.

- **Railways:** these can be extremely hazardous and entering a live track can cause fatalities, so you must always confirm with the emergency services that the rail line is safe to enter before proceeding onto the track to treat a casualty.

- **Location:** there are many ways in which the location of the casualty can pose a hazard, including the:
  - size of the space you have to work in
  - steepness of the ground
  - height off the ground
  - conditions underfoot, e.g. wet grassy slopes, snow, ice
  - amount of available light
  - distance from help.

Link

For more detail on safety considerations and the Fire Triangle, see Unit 2, page 99.

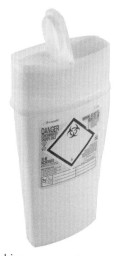

Sharps bin

Link

See page 22 of this unit for more information on PPE.

Link

See page 24 for more information on infection prevention and control (IPC).

Link

See Unit 4, pages 188–89 for more on the effects of poisoning and carbon monoxide.

▶ **Weapons:** where weapons are known to be involved, you should only be present as a first responder once the police deem it safe to do so. First responders may be present where this is required in a different professional capacity, e.g. security staff. When you are conducting your scene survey, note any weapons (or items that can be used as a weapon) that are close to the casualty. Depending on the situation, think about removing these, where you position yourself or withdrawing from the scene and summoning assistance.

▶ **Terrorism:** this remains a real threat to public safety all around the world. Vigilance is required at all times and any suspicious activity should be reported to the police.

▶ **Hazardous material and CBRN incidents:** Hazardous materials can be split into two categories: accidental and intentional.
  • **Accidental:** these are generally known as 'Hazmat incidents'. You should identify the material where possible, e.g. a road tanker will have an information plate (an ADR or Kemler panel) on the side (or back) with some information as to what the load is carrying; bottles of chemicals may have identifying labels. Where possible, pass this information on when summoning assistance.
  • **Intentional:** where there is an intentional release of materials, as in an act of terrorism, these are generally known as CRBN incidents (chemical, radiological, biological, nuclear). You should gather as much information as possible and seek immediate assistance.

▶ **People:** both the casualty's and other people's behaviour (including well-intentioned family and friends) can become a safety hazard at the scene of an incident. Be aware of what people say, how they say it and their body language to determine the hazard they represent. It is these verbal and non-verbal clues that will help to keep you safe.

▶ **Table 1.6**

Verbal cues	Non-verbal cues
▶ Loud speech	▶ Sweating
▶ Shouting	▶ Clenching teeth and jaw
▶ Swearing	▶ Clenched fists
▶ Abusive	▶ Lowering and spreading body
▶ Tone of voice	▶ Staring eyes
	▶ Hand movements
	▶ Standing close
	▶ Aggressive posture
	▶ Facial expression
	▶ Trembling or shaking

Level of risk posed by hazards, and dynamic risk assessment

Level of risk is categorised in two ways:

1 Manageable: a risk that can be removed or reduced to an acceptable level by you within your professional training and scope of practice.

2 Unmanageable: a risk that your professional training and scope of practice does not allow you to attempt to remove or reduce to an acceptable level.

The types of hazards you come across will depend upon your profession and training. For example, entering a burning building as a firefighter will be a manageable risk or dealing with a potentially violent person as a close protection officer will be a manageable risk. It is important to perform a continuous dynamic risk assessment of the hazard and your level of ability to deal with that hazard in order to reduce the risk.

Where there is any doubt, remember the hierarchy of priority and safety:

Self **Other people at the scene** **Casualty**

This may ultimately mean that you must leave the scene having been unable to assess and manage the casualty.

Managing potential conflict and reducing risk

Where there is a potential for conflict, there are a number of measures you can put in place to help keep yourself safe.

▶ Talk to the casualty and be clear about who you are and why you are there. Communicating regularly with the casualty will help to put them at ease.

▶ If you are called to the casualty's property, knock on the door, take a few steps back and give yourself some space.

▶ Ask the casualty to lock away any pets.

▶ Position yourself between the casualty and the exit so you always have a clear exit if needed.

▶ If the casualty is lying on the floor, approach their upper body first, talk to them as you approach so they know you are there and place a hand on their shoulder if they do not respond. If they are lying on their side, place your hand on their uppermost shoulder while approaching from the back. This gives you an element of control and the ability to retreat quickly should they become aggressive.

▶ When in a building and the casualty opens the door, follow them into the property rather than allowing them to close the door behind you. This has a few advantages: you know the exit is unlocked, you are positioned between the exit and the casualty and the casualty will turn their back to you and walk away.
  • Do not allow the casualty to lock the door behind you.
  • Use equipment as a barrier: place this between yourself and the casualty as this will create an obstacle should they approach.

▶ Ask the casualty to sit down; this will make it harder for them to be aggressive towards you.

▶ Request police assistance.

Actions to withdraw from a scene

You need to make a decision based on the level of the threat posed and the situation you are presented with to decide which is the best action to take.

1 Try to give a verbal warning. Explain that if they do not stop their threatening behaviour, you will leave the scene and then be unable to help.

2 Leave the scene and retreat to a safe place.

3 Report this exit, and the hazards with which you were presented, to your control centre.

Quick check

How many hazards can you name that you might encounter as a first responder? Choose three from your list and explain what you would do if confronted by each one.

Personal protective equipment

PPE is any equipment that will protect the user against health or safety risks.

Some of the common PPE items you may have available are shown next.

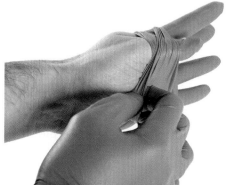

Single-use nitrile gloves provide a barrier when assessing and managing a casualty

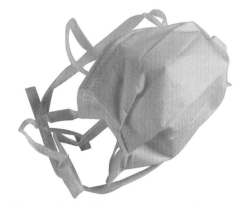

Use a protective face mask to create a barrier where there is potential for infection via particles carried in the air

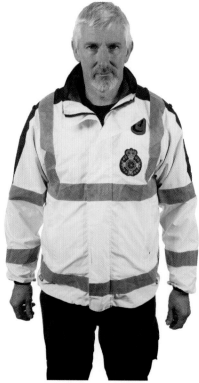

Wear high-visibility clothing to ensure you are easily seen, e.g. when attending roadside incidents

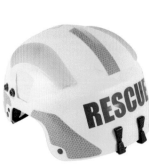

If there is a risk from falling/low objects, you must wear a helmet. If entering a vehicle following a collision, you must wear a helmet.

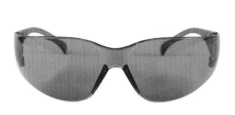
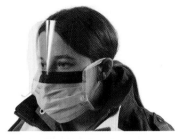

Wear eye protection if there is a risk of splashes or foreign bodies entering the eyes

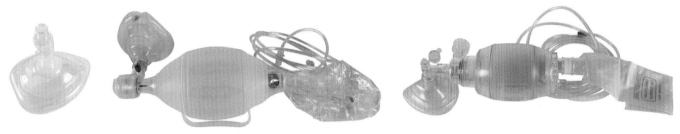

Ear defenders protect your hearing in loud environments

Resuscitation aids (pocket mask and bag-valve-mask) help prevent cross-contamination during resuscitation efforts

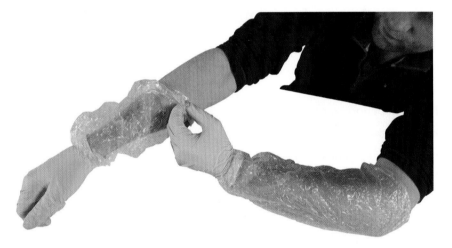
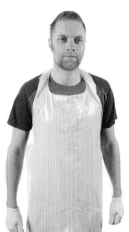

Disposable over-sleeves protect your arms where there is a chance of infection

Disposable aprons protect you from infection

In addition, protective footwear should have solid toe-caps and a good sole to protect your feet.

Assessment practice 1.3   (C, EC) 3.1, 3.3

Claire is giving a presentation to a local group about the hazards she may encounter while working as a first responder.

1 Make a list of the 15 hazards that Claire needs to include in her presentation.

2 Claire wants to create a slide called 'dynamic risk assessment'. What information should she include to explain this?

3 Claire brings in her PPE for the presentation. The group ask her to explain the function of three of the pieces of equipment and to give examples of where she would use them. They choose: gloves, helmet and eye protection. What key points should Claire make sure she covers?

Plan
What information do I need to complete the task?
Where will I find that information?

Do
Place yourself in Claire's position.
What would you do and say?

Review
Have I included as much detail as I can?

Understand the principles relating to infection prevention and control

Knowledge of infection prevention and control (IPC) are vital to your role as a first responder. It will help keep you, your family and your casualties safe from infection.

Your roles and responsibilities

Within your role as a first responder, you will be expected to:

▸ follow universal precautions: good hand hygiene, using correct PPE, safe disposal of waste

▸ use clean equipment only: this is your responsibility

▸ report any possible hazards: you should ensure any hazards are reported to your employer so they are able to manage those hazards

▸ report any potential incidents of infection to your employer

▸ comply with any local IPC laws and regulations.

Employer roles and responsibilities

Your employer is expected to:

▸ comply with any local IPC laws and regulations

▸ provide training to employees

▸ monitor staff performance

▸ monitor the staff working environment

▸ monitor the equipment staff use to ensure it remains fit for purpose

▸ report infection to the health and safety executive where appropriate

▸ provide staff with the correct PPE.

Maintaining professional standards of personal hygiene

It is important that you maintain high standards of personal hygiene. This not only exhibits a professional image to the casualty but also helps to prevent the spread of infection. By giving a professional impression to the casualty you instil confidence. You should have:

▸ clean and tidy nails

▸ clean and tied up or short hair

▸ clean and pressed clothing or uniform

▸ good oral hygiene

▸ any cuts and abrasions covered.

Hand hygiene

Hand hygiene is vital to ensure good IPC. There are five opportunities for cleaning your hands. These are sometimes referred to as the 'five moments for hand hygiene'.

1 before casualty contact

2 before a clean procedure

3 after being exposed to bodily fluids

4 after casualty contact

5 after touching casualty surroundings.

Hand-washing technique using soap and water

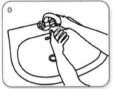
Wet hands with water

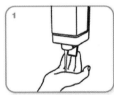
Apply enough soap to cover all hand surfaces

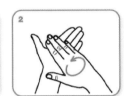
Rub hands palm to palm

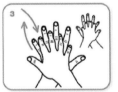
Right palm over left **dorsum** with interlaced fingers and vice versa

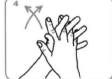
Palm to palm with fingers interlaced

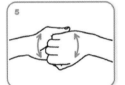
Backs of fingers to opposing palms with fingers interlocked

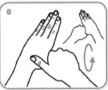
Rotational rubbing of left thumb clasped in right palm and vice versa

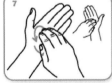
Rotational rubbing, backwards and forwards with clasped fingers of right hand in left

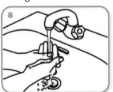
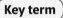
Rinse hands with water

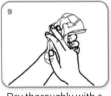
Dry thoroughly with a single-use towel

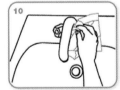
Use towel to turn off tap

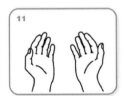
Your hands are safe

Figure 1.4 Hand-washing technique

> **Quick tip**
>
> Use sanitising hand gel if running water is unavailable. It is only effective on hands that are free from any visible particles. It should therefore only be applied once any visible debris has been removed. When you are using hand gel you should use the same technique for rubbing your hands together as if you were using soap and water.

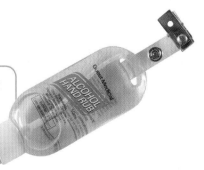

Types of infection

The common transmittable infections you are likely to come across and which can be passed on to you as the first person on scene can be split into four different categories.

▶ **Table 1.7**

Type	Examples	Signs	Symptoms	PPE
Gastroenteritis	▶ Gastroenteritis ▶ Norovirus	▶ Vomiting ▶ Loose stools ▶ Fever	▶ Nausea ▶ Loss of appetite	▶ Gloves ▶ Face mask ▶ Apron
Blood-borne	▶ Hepatitis ▶ HIV	▶ Rapid weight loss ▶ Fever ▶ Prolonged swelling of glands	▶ Extreme and unexplained tiredness, weakness, joint pain	▶ Gloves ▶ Eye protection ▶ Apron
Respiratory	▶ Influenza ▶ Respiratory tract infections	▶ Runny nose ▶ Cough	▶ Congestion ▶ Body aches ▶ Sore throat	▶ Gloves ▶ Face mask
Skin	▶ MRSA	▶ Redness or swelling of skin ▶ Sores ▶ Boils ▶ Swelling	▶ Pain	▶ Gloves

Quick check

What are the steps you need to take to ensure your hands are washed correctly?

Chain of infection

It is important to understand how infections are passed from one person to another (see **Figure 1.5**). Knowledge of IPC breaks this chain to prevent this from happening. It is also important to select the appropriate PPE in order to minimise the risk of you or others contracting infections.

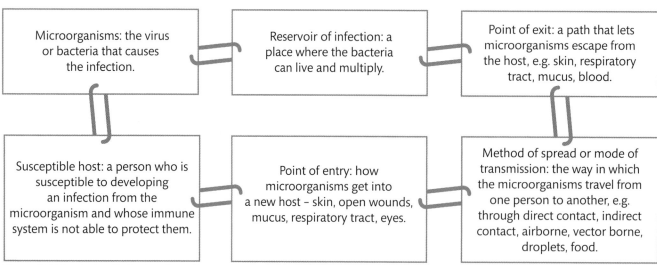

Figure 1.5 The chain of infection shows how infection is passed from person to person

Assessment practice 1.4	(C, EC) 4.3, 4.4

Nic runs his own business providing care to the elderly in the community. He wants to reduce his employees' sick leave by promoting good hygiene. He asks you to produce some information that he can give his employees.

1 A video or poster that explains the correct method for washing hands.

2 A video or poster that explains the chain of infection and how it can be broken at different stages to ensure infection does not spread.

Plan

What key points do I need to get across?
How am I going to produce the end product?
Am I going to create a poster or a video? Maybe use your mobile phone to make a recording.

Do

Gather all of the information and work out the order in which this best conveys the message.

Review

Have I given enough information to the user to be able to complete all of the steps?
Have I explained myself well enough?

Understand the safeguarding of children and vulnerable adults

Safeguarding

It is important that you are able to identify where there is a possible safeguarding issue. You need to be able to identify the signs of abuse and be able to react to these accordingly.

Forms of abuse

Abuse can take many forms and it is important to maintain an open mind when considering if a casualty may be suffering from abuse. To be able to recognise abuse you must be aware of the signs of the different types. While the following list is not exhaustive, it does give details of some examples of the potential signs you may encounter while conducting your duties as a first responder.

▶ Table 1.8

Forms of abuse	Signs of potential abuse
Physical ▶ Assault, such as hitting, slapping, punching, hair pulling ▶ Rough handling ▶ Burns and scalds ▶ Physical punishment ▶ Inappropriate restraint	▶ Series of unexplained falls or major injuries ▶ Injuries/bruising at different stages of healing ▶ Abrasions ▶ Teeth indentations ▶ Injuries to head/face ▶ Casualty may be passive ▶ Bruising in unusual sites, e.g. inner arms and inner thighs ▶ Finger pattern bruising ▶ Injuries not matching with account of what happened

▶ **Table 1.8** continued

Forms of abuse	Signs of potential abuse
Sexual ▶ Rape ▶ Sexual assault ▶ Inappropriate touching ▶ Sexual photography ▶ Indecent exposure	▶ Change in behaviour ▶ Overt sexual behaviour or language ▶ Difficulty in walking/sitting ▶ Injuries to genital/anal area ▶ Bruising ▶ Foreign bodies in genital or anal openings ▶ Self harm ▶ Reluctance to be alone with a particular person
Psychological or emotional ▶ Threats ▶ Denying privacy ▶ Enforcing social isolation ▶ Preventing someone from making their own choices ▶ Intimidation ▶ Harassment ▶ Bullying ▶ Verbal abuse	▶ Withdrawn ▶ Depression ▶ Cowering and fearfulness ▶ Change in sleep patterns ▶ Agitation ▶ Confusion ▶ Change in behaviours ▶ Change in appetite/weight ▶ Looking towards others to make their decisions ▶ Low self esteem ▶ Lack of communication when a particular person is present
Financial ▶ Theft of money ▶ Fraud ▶ Preventing someone from accessing their own money ▶ Exploiting a person's resources, e.g. eating their food without consent ▶ Arranging less care than is needed to maximise their own inheritance	▶ Unexplained unpaid bills ▶ Basic needs not being met ▶ Lack of cash on a day-to-day basis ▶ Missing possessions ▶ Unnecessary property repairs ▶ Disparity between living conditions and their financial resources
Institutional ▶ Rigid regimes ▶ Insufficient staff ▶ Not providing adequate food and drink ▶ Lack of dignity	▶ Poor care standards ▶ Lack of positive response to complex needs ▶ Rigid routines ▶ Inadequate staffing ▶ Insufficient knowledge base ▶ Public discussion of personal matters ▶ Absence of individual care plans
Neglect and self-neglect ▶ Failure to administer medication ▶ Failure to allow access to basic needs ▶ Providing care in a way that the person dislikes ▶ Lack of self care ▶ Inability to manage personal affairs	▶ Failure to meet basic needs ▶ No access to services ▶ Isolation ▶ Absence of prescribed medication ▶ Poor environment ▶ Accumulation of untaken medication

Quick check

Can you give five examples of physical abuse and list the signs and symptoms that you may see?

When abuse is suspected

`6 Steps`

1 You have a duty to report suspected abuse. You should follow your local guidelines for how, and to whom, this report should be made.

2 Consider if you need to summon the police to protect the person immediately or to help remove the casualty to the ambulance to treat them.

3 It is good practice to make a note of your concerns as soon as possible after the event, including what has happened and any action you have taken. This is to ensure you do not miss any details.

4 Your role is not to investigate the situation or confront the person thought responsible for the abuse, as any such action could jeopardise the situation and affect action taken subsequently.

5 It is important to identify and note any potential sources of evidence. Ensure you include this in your report, informing the clinician when you hand over the care of the casualty and any police officers who have been made aware of the situation.

6 Relay your concerns to the next echelon of care as soon as possible. This is important for the casualty's continuation of care and, as a result, the clinical team may identify more signs during their assessment. Do this in complete confidence. You may need to make an excuse to speak to the clinician privately away from the casualty and other bystanders.

When abuse is disclosed

`8 Steps`

1 You have a duty to report suspected abuse where it is disclosed. You should follow your local guidelines for how, and to whom, this report should be made. You may have to complete a referral to your organisation's safeguarding officer as well as the local social services.

2 People may ask you not to tell anyone about the abuse. They may say 'I need to tell you something but you won't say anything, will you?' You need to make it clear that you may have to make a confidential report to other agencies depending on what they tell you. Do not promise the casualty anything. Instead, assure them that you will only share information with relevant agencies if necessary.

3 Listening to the casualty carefully and making them feel they are heard and believed is extremely important. Do not question the casualty about the disclosure as this falls outside of your role. Instead, offer support and show the casualty that you care.

4 Ensure the immediate safety of the casualty. If they have become ill or injured, manage the symptoms and ensure that you inform the next echelon of care when you hand over the casualty.

5 Inform the police and ask them to attend where it appears there has been a criminal offence.

6 Preserve evidence where possible. For example, if you suspect the casualty has been sexually assaulted and they give you items of clothing to dispose of, keep them in a clean bag for the police.

continued on page 30

When abuse is disclosed (*continued*)

7 Record all the details of the concerns clearly and factually as soon as possible after disclosure and ensure that the next echelon of clinical care is made aware of your concerns.

8 Any physical injuries should be recorded on a PRF.

Assessment practice 1.5 (C, EC) 5.1

Bella has started to work as a first responder and she is completing some training provided by her employer relating to safeguarding. She has been asked to complete the following table by listing as many different types of abuse that she can remember. She has come to you for some help.

▶ **Table 1.9**

Type of abuse	Examples	Signs of abuse

Plan

How many different types of abuse should I include?

Do

Try and complete the table from memory without looking back at the information in the book.

Review

Compare your table with the answers in this unit to see what you have missed.

Understand post-incident procedures

Effective clinical handover

Following your assessment and management of the casualty you may need to hand over clinician responsibility to the next echelon of care. This may be someone within your organisation who has a qualification at a higher level than your own or it may be to the local ambulance service. It is important to ensure that you pass on detailed information about the incident and the casualty in a precise and succinct manner. Your handover must include:

▶ name, sex and age of the casualty

▶ details of what happened

▶ details of when the incident happened

▶ details of the injuries you have seen or suspected

▶ the casualty's vital signs

▶ details of the management you have given.

Three of the most common ways to structure your handover for the next echelon of care are listed next. These are provided as mnemonic acronyms to help you remember each piece of information to include in your handover.

ATMIST

▶ **A**ge and sex of the casualty

▶ **T**ime of the incident

▶ **M**echanism of injury

> **Quick tip**
>
> Completing an ATMIST handover should take no more than 60 seconds.

> **Quick tip**
>
> ATMIST may differ between trauma and medical patients.

▸ **I**njuries seen or suspected

▸ **S**igns – vital signs/observations of the casualty including heart rate, respiration rate, consciousness level and any changes seen in these

▸ **T**reatment – any management you have given the casualty.

ASHICE

▸ **A**ge of casualty

▸ **S**ex of casualty

▸ **H**istory – the cause of the injury or illness

▸ **I**njuries or illness – how is the casualty injured or what signs and symptoms of illness have been presented?

▸ **C**ondition – vital signs/observations of the casualty including heart rate, respiration rate, consciousness level and any changes seen in these

▸ **E**stimated time of arrival at hospital; some providers use this E as 'Everything else' and include anything else that is important to the casualty's management.

SBAR

▸ **S**ituation – casualty identification, plus who you are and the nature of your role

▸ **B**ackground – past medical history, history about what has happened

▸ **A**ssessment – vital signs and symptoms reported

▸ **R**ecommendation – what help you need and what stage you have reached in the management of the casualty.

Patient Report Form

A PRF should be completed as a permanent record of the incident you have attended. Your organisation should provide you with these and they must be completed for every incident. They form part of the records for that casualty and, where practicable, a copy should accompany the casualty when they are handed over to the next level of care. A copy should be retained by the organisation as a record of what has occurred. While each PRF will have a different appearance, there are many common components.

Components of a PRF

▸ casualty demographics, i.e. name, age, date of birth, address

▸ location of incident

▸ primary survey findings

▸ history of presenting complaint – what exactly happened leading up to the injury or illness?

▸ 'on arrival' – what you found when you arrived at the scene (position, movement and normal/abnormal skin colour of casualty)

▸ 'on examination' (signs and symptoms, **pertinent negatives**)

▸ capacity

▸ social history, e.g. smoker, alcohol intake, housing, recent foreign travel

▸ past medical history

▸ family past medical history

Quick tip

Remember that the completed PRF is a confidential document. You should also exercise caution when using photography to gather mechanism of injury evidence.

Link

See Unit 2, page 42 for more information on the primary survey.

Key term

Pertinent negative – relevant information that would help to rule out any conditions, e.g. no vomiting, no chest pain.

- vital signs (initial set and during periodic reassessment) of the casualty including heart rate, respiration rate, consciousness level etc.
- allergies
- treatment given – what you have done to manage the casualty.

Date: 1st April 2017	Time: 13:40	Job Number: 023

Casualty Name: Roxanne Gunn	Date of Birth: 12th November 1994	Age: 22	Gender: Female

Home Address: 10 Coronation Street, Blackpool, BL1 1BL

Incident Location: Blackpool Beach

History of Presenting Complaint: Casualty was running on the beach when she started to feel some chest tightness and was struggling to catch her breath. She sat down and one of the event marshals called for assistance

Consent given: yes		Capacity: yes
Past Medical History: Asthma Irritable bowel syndrome Hayfever	**Medications:** Salbutamol	**Family Past Medical History** Grandmother has asthma

Social History: Lives at home with sister and parents, student, non-smoker, no alcohol, no recent foreign travel.	**Allergies:** Dust, Pollen

Primary Survey: No catastrophic haemorrhage, alert and orientated. A – open, clear and patent. B – 28 regular, C – 110, Strong regular pulse.

On arrival: Casualty sat on a chair, leaning forward, Short of breath, fully alert and orientated, no pale, no cyanosis.

On Examination:

A – Open, clear and patent

B – 28 regular with equal rise and fall of the chest, tachypnoea, short of breath at rest, non-productive cough, unable to speak in complete sentences, accessory muscle use, leaning forward in chair, appears visibly distressed. Some chest tightness, no pain on respiration.

C – 110 strong and regular radial pulse, tachycardic, no cardiac chest pain, no palpitations, skin warm and dry to touch, cap refill < 2 seconds, not pale, no nausea, no vomiting.

D – alert on AVPU, no confusion, fast negative   E – fully mobile, no pain, says she feels cool

Vital signs:

Time	13:40	13:50	14:00	14:15					
RR	28	28	20	16					
HR	110	108	100	98					
AVPU	A	A	A	A					
SpO$_2$	96%	99%	100%	100%					
Pupil size	2 / 2	2 / 2	2 / 2	2 / 2					
Pain score	1	1	0	0					

Management: Calmed and reassured casualty, asked marshal to collect casualty's medication, encouraged casualty to take medication as prescribed by GP, warmed casualty with blankets. Following taking medication x 4 doses, casualty's breathing improved. Respiration rate reduced and she began to feel much better, she was then able to speak in full sentences with no accessory muscle use. Casualty's dad was at the race and she was left with him, he was happy to monitor and she will speak to her GP tomorrow as these episodes are happening more often.

Handover to: Left in the care of father	Handover Time: 14:15

Casualty Signature: *Roxie Gunn*	Date: 1 / 4 / 17

First Responder Signature: Susan Mansfield	Date: 1 / 4 / 17

Figure 1.6 Example of a completed PRF

Ensuring equipment is serviceable and available post-incident

Following the completion of an incident you need to ensure that the equipment is ready for the next occasion. The equipment that you have used can be split into two categories:

1 disposable, e.g. single-use nitrile gloves, single-use face shield

2 reusable, e.g. protective footwear, eye protection, pulse oximetry.

Disposable items or reusable items that are unable to be sufficiently cleaned should be disposed of appropriately in one of three ways:

1 General waste – black bag. This should include any items that do not contain bodily fluids, e.g. packaging.

2 Clinical waste – yellow or orange bag. This should include any materials that contain any bodily fluids, e.g. dressings containing blood.

3 Sharps bin – yellow bin. This is secure for any sharp items that have been used. Any used sharps, such as a lancet used to check a casualty's blood sugars levels, should be placed immediately into the bin after their use.

Clean reusable items with an appropriate disinfectant wipe. Any item that is either visibly soiled or has had direct casualty contact should be cleaned and placed back into its normal place ready for the next casualty.

It is your responsibility to ensure your equipment is ready for the next casualty. This means you will have to replace and restock any of the equipment you have discarded.

You should wear clean and freshly laundered uniform for each shift. Carefully remove any uniform that is soiled with bodily fluids and change into clean uniform. If you need to pass soiled uniform over your head, for example a T-shirt, you may need to cut this off instead to avoid contact with the soiled material and your face. Place soiled uniform in a **soluble bag**, then wash at the highest temperature allowed for the garment. Tumble drying or ironing will further help to reduce the chance of infection. It is useful to have clean uniform easily accessible.

Your mental health

Your own mental wellbeing can be affected by the scenes and casualties that you deal with while performing your role as a first responder. Research has suggested that members of the emergency services are at risk of developing a mental health problem.

You have good mental wellbeing if you:

▶ have strong relationships with others

▶ have a good level of self esteem

▶ feel relatively confident

▶ feel content

▶ feel productive at work

▶ cope well with daily stresses

▶ are able to express your emotions.

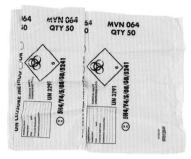
Clinical waste bags

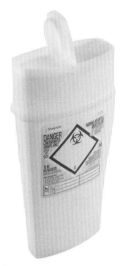
Sharps bin

> **Key term**
>
> **Soluble bag** – a special bag that can be placed directly into a washing machine where the seams of the bag are destroyed by the water to allow the clothes to be washed without handling them.

When to seek help

You should seek help:

▶ when experiencing prolonged negative feelings that contradict any of the indicators of good mental wellbeing

▶ when experiencing, or when others comment that they have noticed, prolonged signs or symptoms of:
  • depression
  • anxiety
  • post-traumatic stress disorder.

Available support

Support is available to you but taking those first steps to seek it can be hard. Your own General Practitioner (GP) could be your first point of contact. Discuss your thoughts and feelings with the GP, who can refer you for more specialist help where required. Some organisations also have an internal programme of support and you may be able to access these – they are normally staffed by trained colleagues who are available to help and support you.

If you do not feel comfortable talking to your GP or you want to learn more about mental health, there is information available from other organisations. Even if you feel well, it is worth investigating some of these organisations for support material:

▶ MIND Blue Light Programme

▶ Blue Lamp Foundation.

Assessment practice 1.6 (C, EC) 6.1, 6.2

It is a cold November Wednesday evening at approximately 18.45 when you attend a road traffic collision where a push bike has been struck by a car as it was going around a roundabout. The cyclist was wearing a helmet and witnesses say he did not talk to them for a short time – although he is now sitting on the pavement, a little confused.

The casualty, Joe, is trying to get fit since being diagnosed with diabetes last month just before his 60th birthday. He cannot recall exactly what has happened but his helmet is broken and there is a circular crack on the car windscreen. He is breathing normally at a rate of 16 breaths per minute, has a strong regular radial pulse at 90 beats per minute and is alert and orientated. He is able to talk to you normally. You clean and dry a small cut on Joe's nose. Joe also has pain in his right wrist that he gives a score of 5 out of 10. You bandage this accordingly. He says he has no other pain but you ask him to stay still anyway until help arrives. A paramedic in a rapid response car pulls up and she walks towards you.

1 Use ATMIST to give her a handover.

2 Complete a PRF for this incident.

Plan

What is the information I must give the paramedic?

What information can I use to complete my PRF? Highlight the important parts.

Do

Use the information from the text to give a handover in less than 60 seconds. Practise reading this out so you get used to doing this verbally.

Review

Ask someone else on your course to review your PRF to see if you have missed anything.

Further reading and resources

www.mind.org.uk

www.nspcc.org.uk

www.nice.org.uk

www.infectionpreventioncontrol.co.uk

www.bluelamp-foundation.org

www.hse.gov.uk/guidance/

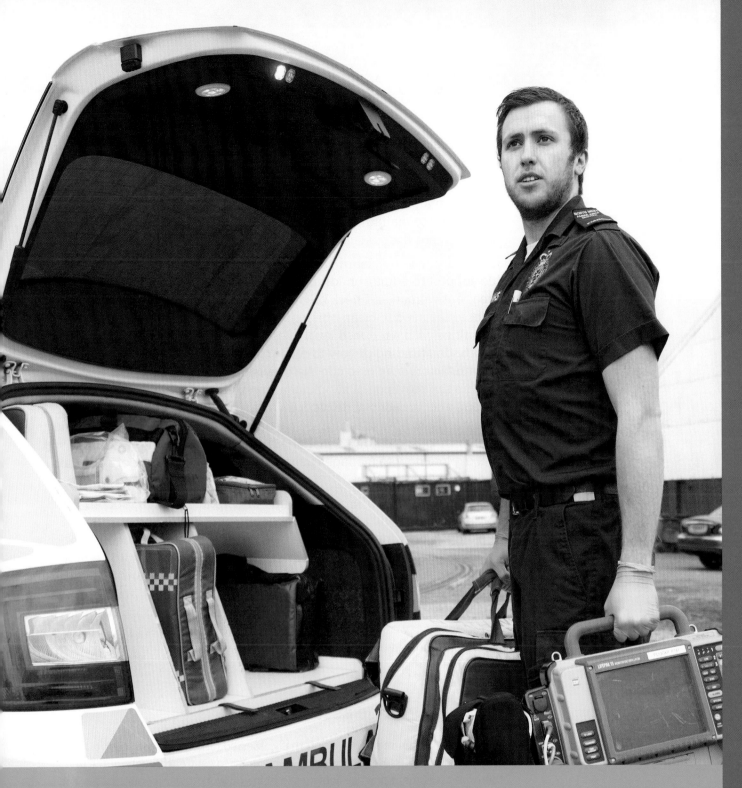

Emergency Care of Casualties for the First Responder

2

Getting to know your unit

Understanding how to manage casualties with life-threatening injuries or illnesses is vital for all care providers from first aiders to registered healthcare professionals. The primary survey is designed to quickly identify the risk posed to life and inform your decision making in terms of the casualty's management needs so that you can act swiftly and confidently to maintain life in the critical moments before the arrival of definitive pre-hospital care.

In this unit you will learn about the key principles of providing basic life support to adults, children, infants and special casualties such as pregnant women and neck breathers. You will also learn about the techniques used to clear, open, maintain and manage the airway of casualties with a reduced level of consciousness. You will develop your understanding of how to recognise and manage situations where certain factors may preclude the provision of life support. You will explore the provision of supplementary oxygen, including the correct dosage and methods of delivery for a range of casualties. You will go on to learn about how to recognise casualties suffering from catastrophic haemorrhages and how to manage these using tourniquets. Finally, you will explore how to manage casualties choking as a result of both mild and severe obstructions.

You will develop your knowledge and understanding in a theoretical context and you will also, in a simulated environment, practically explore the principles and techniques used by the first responder to assess casualties and provide initial emergency care. This will enable you to develop specific skills for assessment within this unit but will also prepare you for the final synoptic unit in which your ability to competently manage incidents involving a wide range of casualties who require primary and continuing assessment, basic life support and other aspects of emergency care covered in this unit.

How you will be assessed

This unit will comprise a series of internally assessed tasks set by your centre. How they perform this assessment will vary from centre to centre. Throughout the unit there are assessment practice activities to help you work towards your assessment. Completing these will not mean that you have achieved a Pass or Fail, but that you have carried out useful research and preparation.

In order to achieve a Pass, you need to meet all the Assessment criteria. The assessment set by your centre will consist of a number of tasks designed to meet the criteria in the following tables. This may include activities such as:

▶ creating a written report about the process of assessing casualties using the correct processes

▶ creating a report about the provision of basic life support including modifications for special casualties

▶ producing a video guide demonstrating elements of basic life support provision.

How the unit is covered: In order to ensure the content follows a logical procedural progression of care, the order in the coverage of the Learning outcomes and Assessment criteria may differ from those shown next. All LOs and ACs are, however, covered in the unit.

Unit 2 Learning outcomes and Assessment criteria (Certificate)

▶ **Table 2.1**

Learning outcome 1: Understand the assessment of conscious and unconscious casualties

Assessment criteria	
1.1	Explain the process of assessing casualties using the DRCA(c)BCDE protocol
1.2	Explain the circumstances in which the pulse is not used to assess the presence of circulation in the primary survey

Learning outcome 2: Explore the principles of basic life support for adults, children and infants

Assessment criteria	
2.1	Explain the principles of basic life support for adults
2.2	Explain the use of an automated external defibrillator
2.3	Demonstrate the use of four different methods of providing rescue breaths to an adult
2.4	Demonstrate the use of mouth-to-mouth-and-nose ventilation for providing rescue breaths to an infant
2.5	Explain the modifications to the protocols basic life support for special casualties
2.6	Explain the role of the Advanced Decision and DNA-CPRs in basic life support

Learning outcome 3: Explore the techniques used to manage the airway of casualties with a reduced level of consciousness

Assessment criteria	
3.1	Explain the different techniques used to clear an airway for adults, children and infants with a reduced level of consciousness
3.2	Demonstrate the use of postural drainage to clear an airway for a casualty with a reduced level of consciousness
3.3	Demonstrate the use of suction to clear an airway for a casualty with a reduced level of consciousness
3.4	Demonstrate the use of a single finger sweep to remove a visible object from the airway for a child or infant
3.5	Explain the different techniques to open an airway for adults, children and infants with a reduced level of consciousness
3.6	Demonstrate the use of the head tilt and chin lift to open an airway for an adult, child or infant with a reduced level of consciousness
3.7	Demonstrate the use of the neutral alignment to open an airway for an infant with a reduced level of consciousness
3.8	Demonstrate the use of the jaw thrust to open an airway for an adult, child or infant with a reduced level of consciousness
3.9	Explain the use of different techniques to maintain the open airway for adults, children and infants with a reduced level of consciousness
3.10	Demonstrate the use of the safe airway position to maintain the open airway of an adult, child or infant with a reduced level of consciousness
3.11	Demonstrate the use of airway adjuncts to maintain the open airway of adults with reduced levels of consciousness
3.12	Demonstrate the use of airway adjuncts to maintain the open airway of children with reduced levels of consciousness
3.13	Demonstrate the use of airway adjuncts to maintain the open airway of infants with reduced levels of consciousness

Learning outcome 4: Understand the recognition and management of life extinct

Assessment criteria	
4.1	Describe the recognition factors for determining life extinct
4.2	Explain actions to be taken following the establishment of life extinct

Learning outcome 5: Explore the provision of supplementary oxygen

Assessment criteria	
5.1	Explain how to select the correct method and flow rate for delivering supplemental oxygen for four different types of casualty
5.2	Demonstrate how to safely configure an oxygen system for use
5.3	Demonstrate how to administer supplemental oxygen using four different oxygen supplementation delivery devices

Learning outcome 6: Explore the recognition and management of a casualty with a catastrophic haemorrhage

Assessment criteria	
6.1	Describe what is meant by the term catastrophic haemorrhage
6.2	Explain the management of a casualty with a catastrophic limb haemorrhage
6.3	Demonstrate the use of a tourniquet to control a catastrophic limb haemorrhage

Learning outcome 7: Explore the techniques used to manage choking casualties

Assessment criteria	
7.1	Explain the process of recognising and managing a conscious choking casualty
7.2	Demonstrate the management of a conscious choking adult or child
7.3	Demonstrate the management of a conscious choking infant

Unit 2 Learning outcomes and Assessment criteria (Extended Certificate)

▶ **Table 2.2**

Learning outcome 1: Understand the assessment of conscious and unconscious casualties

Assessment criteria	
1.1	Explain the process of assessing casualties using the DRCA(c)BCDE protocol
1.2	Explain the circumstances in which the pulse is not routinely used to assess the presence of circulation in the primary survey

Learning outcome 2: Explore the principles of basic life support for adults, children and infants

Assessment criteria	
2.1	Explain the principles of basic life support for adults
2.2	Explain the use of an automated external defibrillator
2.3	Demonstrate the use of four different methods of providing rescue breaths to an adult
2.4	Demonstrate the use of mouth-to-mouth-and-nose ventilation for providing rescue breaths to an infant
2.5	Explain the modifications to the protocols basic life support for special casualties
2.6	Explain the role of the Advanced Decision and DNA-CPRs in basic life support

Learning outcome 3: Explore the techniques used to manage the airway of casualties with a reduced level of consciousness

	Assessment criteria
3.1	Explain the different techniques used to clear an airway for adults, children and infants with a reduced level of consciousness
3.2	Demonstrate the use of postural drainage to clear an airway for a casualty with a reduced level of consciousness
3.3	Demonstrate the use of suction to clear an airway for a casualty with a reduced level of consciousness
3.4	Demonstrate the use of a single finger sweep to remove a visible object from the airway for a child or infant with a reduced level of consciousness
3.5	Explain the different techniques to open an airway for adults, children and infants with a reduced levels of consciousness
3.6	Demonstrate the use of the head tilt and chin lift to open an airway for an adult, child or infant with a reduced level of consciousness
3.7	Demonstrate the use of the neutral alignment to open an airway for an infant with a reduced level of consciousness
3.8	Demonstrate the use of the jaw thrust to open an airway for an adult, child or infant with a reduced level of consciousness
3.9	Explain the use of different techniques to maintain the open airway for adults, children and infants with a reduced level of consciousness
3.10	Demonstrate the use of the safe airway position to maintain the open airway of an adult, child or infant with a reduced level of consciousness
3.11	Demonstrate the use of airway adjuncts to maintain the open airway of adults with reduced levels of consciousness
3.12	Demonstrate the use of airway adjuncts to maintain the open airway of children with reduced levels of consciousness
3.13	Demonstrate the use of airway adjuncts to maintain the open airway of infants with reduced levels of consciousness

Learning outcome 4: Understand the recognition and management of life extinct

	Assessment criteria
4.1	Describe the recognition factors for determining life extinct
4.2	Explain actions to be taken following the establishment of life extinct

Learning outcome 5: Explore the provision of supplementary oxygen

	Assessment criteria
5.1	Explain how to select the correct method and flow rate for delivering supplemental oxygen for four different types of casualty
5.2	Demonstrate how to safely configure an oxygen system for use
5.3	Demonstrate how to administer supplemental oxygen using four different oxygen supplementation delivery devices

Learning outcome 6: Explore the recognition and management of a casualty with a catastrophic haemorrhage

Assessment criteria	
6.1	Describe what is meant by the term catastrophic haemorrhage
6.2	Explain the management of a casualty with a catastrophic haemorrhage
6.3	Demonstrate the use of a tourniquet to control a catastrophic haemorrhage
6.4	Demonstrate wound packing using a haemostatic agent to control a catastrophic junctional haemorrhage

Learning outcome 7: Explore the techniques used to manage choking casualties

Assessment criteria	
7.1	Explain the process of recognising and managing a conscious choking casualty
7.2	Demonstrate the management of a conscious choking adult or child
7.3	Demonstrate the management of a conscious choking infant

Getting started

Work in groups of between four and six people. On slips of paper think of as many injuries or medical emergencies as you can. Discuss how you would prioritise the emergencies and then arrange the slips into the priority of treatment needed. Why have you ordered them in this way?

Still in your groups, consider whether the priority order would be different if you were a First Responder working alone. Think about what you would assess or check in an unconscious casualty, in what order and why?

Understand the assessment of conscious and unconscious casualties

All casualties will be assessed using the following protocol: DRCA(c)BCDE. By following this standardised procedure for all casualties, you will be able to ensure continuity of care among care providers and by following the protocol's hierarchy, you can focus on treatment order and priority.

Casualty assessment protocol

DRCA(c)BCDE

Link

See page 61 for further information on the complexities of checking a pulse.

The ABC (airway, breathing, circulation) protocol was first developed in the 1950s and has since evolved to the larger mnemonic: DRCA(c)BCDE. While almost universal, the terminology varies slightly in different parts of the world or within different organisations, but all variations feature the same hierarchical order and focus on the same ABC protocol as being essential to life.

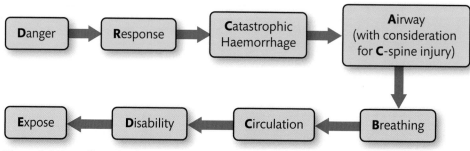

Figure 2.1 You will need to learn and apply this DRCA(c)BCDE protocol

- ▶ The assessment for Danger is a continuation of the scene management.
- ▶ RCABCD is commonly referred to as the **primary survey**. This is a rapid assessment and management of the most immediately life-threatening conditions.
- ▶ 'Expose' is a physical examination for injuries. It is considered a **secondary survey** (sometimes known as the Secondary Assessment).

This procedure is applied to all casualties in all situations. The procedure guides the responder to the most serious potential issues that may not be obvious upon first impression. For example:

- ▶ A seemingly large amount of blood may not, in fact, be the most pressing issue but may distract the responder from a more serious issue, such as a casualty's blocked airway.

Key terms

Primary survey – a systematic assessment of immediately life-threatening issues.

Secondary survey – a systematic assessment of other injuries or evidence of medical conditions.

▶ A conscious, vocal casualty with obvious injuries may distract the responder from less obvious dangers at the scene.

Applying a standardised procedure not only ensures continuity of care for all casualties, but also provides objective guidance towards the casualty's treatment needs.

Danger

In Unit 1 you learned about the importance of recognising dangers at the scene to yourself, other people and the casualty. Before any casualty is approached, assessed and treated, all dangers should be removed or reduced to a reasonably safe level.

Response

Rather than looking to see if the casualty is simply conscious or unconscious you must examine their **level of response**. What are they able to respond to and how do they respond?

▶ **Table 2.3**

1 **A**lert	The casualty is fully orientated in place, time and person: they know who they are, where they are, and they are aware of their surroundings. They will also be replying clearly and appropriately.
2 Responding to **V**oice	The casualty is able to respond, in some way to verbal stimuli.
3 Responding to **P**ain	The casualty is able to respond, in some way to painful stimuli.
4 **U**nresponsive	The casualty is unable to respond to any stimuli.

It is important to note that:

▶ a casualty's level of response is not determined by whether their eyes are open or closed or whether they are standing up or lying down, it is determined by their ability to respond

▶ any response is a valid response, whether it is an overt, obvious response such as opening their eyes and looking at you or a subtle response such as a flickering of the eyes or a flinch.

Link

For more information on scene management, see Unit 1, page 14.

Key term

Level of response – a system to measure and record a casualty's level of consciousness based on their ability to respond to different stimuli.

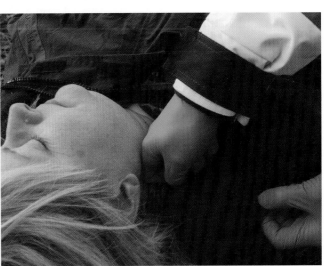

Check the casualty's response to voice

Check the casualty's response to pain

How to assess a casualty's level of response

▸ If the casualty appears conscious, talk to them. How they respond will determine whether they are fully alert (i.e. speaking clearly and appropriately) or simply responding to voice (i.e. mumbling or slurring their words).

▸ If the casualty appears unconscious, talk to them as you approach. In the first instance, ask them a question such as 'Can you tell me what happened?'. This is a better question than 'Can you hear me?' as it requires greater **cognitive ability** to understand and answer. It may also elicit a better quality reply than a simple 'Yes' or 'No'. Information offered by the casualty is of as much value as how they are able to talk to you.

   • If their reply is clear and appropriate and they seem fully orientated, then they are fully alert. If their response is slurred, confused or incomprehensible, they are responsive to voice.

▸ If the casualty is unable to respond to a question, give a loud, direct command such as 'Open your eyes!'. Regardless of whether their response is overt or subtle, if they are able to respond in any way, they are still considered to be responsive to voice.

▸ If the casualty is unable to respond to any verbal stimuli, administer a measured amount of pain, by applying pressure with a knuckle to the side of the neck. Typically, pain is exhibited in the face with a wince or flinch. Any response seen at this stage would place the casualty as responsive to pain.

▸ If the casualty does not respond to a painful stimulus, they are unresponsive.

Difficulties in assessing response

Applying the AVPU scale can be difficult on some casualties. Casualties with dementia, for example, may never appear fully alert if they suffer with disorientation or their speech typically appears confused. You need to consider what normal behaviour is for them.

Assessing the response of an infant (a year old and below) also presents problems. In this instance you should look for normal behaviour as a sign of being alert.

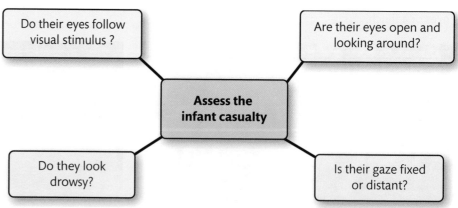

Figure 2.2 Assess the infant casualty

If the infant appears to be asleep, try and rouse them by talking to them. If this is unsuccessful, rather than shouting 'Open your eyes!' as you would to an adult, clap loudly next to their ear to assess their ability to respond to noise.

If this does not elicit a response, administer a small amount of pain by flicking the soles of their feet to see if they respond.

Warning: Never press on the neck of an infant.

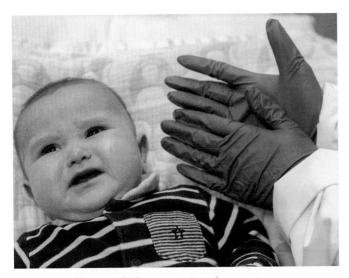
Check the infant casualty's response to noise

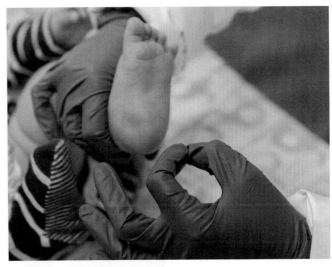
Check the infant casualty's response to pain

Explore the recognition and management of a casualty with a catastrophic haemorrhage

Catastrophic haemorrhage is an event that can be defined as an immediately life-threatening bleed, which is external, compressible and cannot be controlled by direct pressure.

A catastrophic haemorrhage is catastrophic in nature because of the rapid onset of **hypovolaemic shock**, likely to cause death in minutes.

During your initial assessment of the casualty you must consider whether the casualty is in an 'immediately life-threatening' situation. You must look for, and deal with, catastrophic haemorrhage at this stage before you move on to assess anything else.

Gauging blood loss can be extremely difficult: a small amount of blood on a white tiled floor can look serious; conversely a large amount of blood may be lost into sand, gravel or soil and very little of it will be seen. For the purpose of recognising 'immediately life-threatening' bleeding this is actively squirting blood from an artery.

If catastrophic haemorrhage is identified, it should be treated immediately.

Management of catastrophic haemorrhage

The management of catastrophic haemorrhage depends upon whether the wound is on the head, neck or torso, or on a limb only (see **Figure 2.3**).

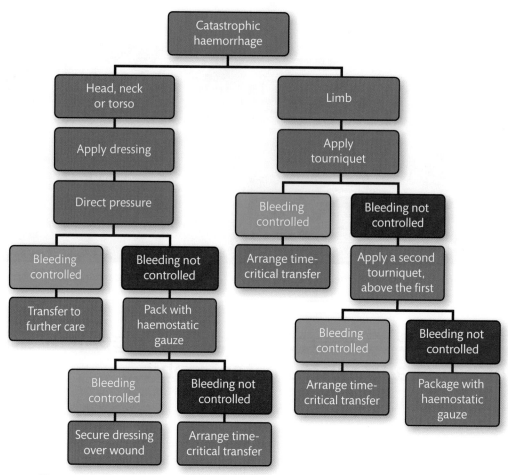

Figure 2.3 Different processes apply depending on the location of the bleeding

Tourniquet use

▸ The first tourniquet is applied above the joint (either knee or elbow).
There is inconclusive evidence as to the effectiveness of placing a tourniquet on a **single or double bone compartment**. For simplicity and continuity, all first tourniquets are placed on a single bone compartment.

▸ The first tourniquet is placed as close to the joint as possible.
There is some evidence to suggest that the tourniquet is most effective when placed in the centre of the thigh or upper arm. The tourniquet is placed close to the joint, however, to preserve as much viable tissue as possible should a surgical amputation be required.

▸ The tourniquet is applied as tightly as possible.
Arterial blood is at a higher pressure than venous blood (from veins); as such, if the tourniquet is not tight enough, bleeding may have stopped but arterial blood is able to enter the limb beyond the tourniquet, while venous blood cannot return out of the limb. This can cause pressure to build in the limb beyond the tourniquet, causing tissue damage – a serious condition called compartment syndrome. Some guidelines suggest the tourniquet should be tightened until a **distal** pulse can no longer be felt. Given the difficulty in detecting a pulse in normal conditions this is not considered to be reliable. For simplicity and continuity, the tourniquet should be tightened past the point at which bleeding is stopped.

Key terms

Single or double bone compartment – a single bone compartment (e.g. the upper arm or thigh) has only one bone. A double bone compartment (e.g. lower leg and lower arm) has two bones.

Distal – away from. In this instance, the end of the limb. The antonym to this is 'proximal'.

Extended Certificate: This requires that you can explain the management of a casualty and tourniquet use with all types of catastrophic haemorrhage. The Certificate covers catastrophic limb haemorrhage and tourniquet use on limbs only.

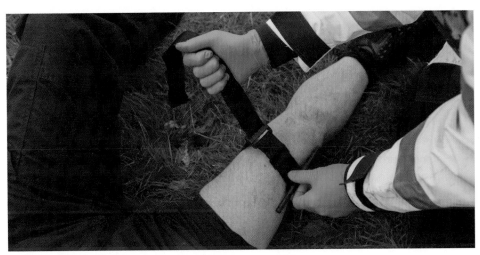

Apply the first tourniquet as close above the joint as possible

▶ If bleeding has not been stopped, apply a second tourniquet above the first. As the first tourniquet has been applied as close to the joint as possible, there is no room available below the first.

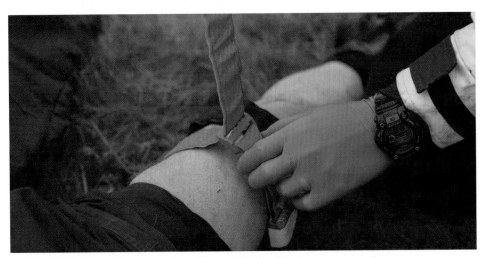

A second tourniquet application should be used if bleeding has not stopped

▶ Mark the time on the tourniquet and on your Patient Report Form (PRF).

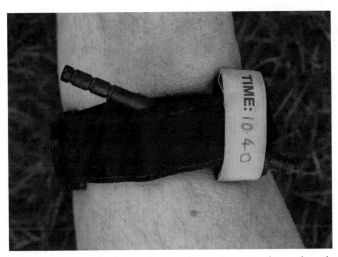

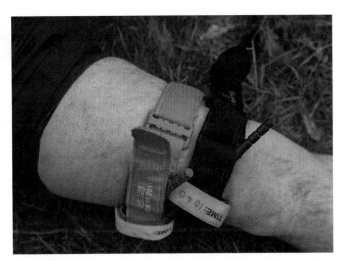

Mark the time on the first and second tourniquets to show when they were applied

Haemostatic agents (Extended Certificate)

▸ Haemostatic agents are dressings designed to promote clotting and arrest catastrophic bleeding. There are several brands of haemostatic agents available and many act in different ways. Different brands of haemostatic agents work in slightly different ways. Familiarise yourself with the brand you will be using.

▸ The gauze must be pushed deep into a **junctional wound** – this may require more than one packet.

▸ Haemostatic agents do not work without direct pressure. Continue to apply direct pressure even when using a haemostatic agent.

If practical, attach the packet to the casualty so that the receiving hospital knows which brand of haemostatic agent has been used. This may help the process of removing the gauze in surgery.

Aftercare

▸ Once the bleeding has stopped, continue through the remainder of the primary survey protocol.

▸ Although the bleeding has been arrested, the casualty needs pre-emptive management to prevent the onset of hypovolaemic shock.

▸ By the application of tourniquets or wound packaging, the casualty has been made time-critical. In a triage situation, any casualty treated for catastrophic haemorrhage is escalated to Category 1; the initial injury has been dealt with but they require definitive hospital care as a priority.
Report the application and time of any tourniquets or wound packing administered at the clinical handover.

▸ Tourniquets remain in place if the transfer to definitive care is less than one hour. If the transfer is more than an hour, seek advice from the receiving hospital.

Airway

With all dangers removed, the casualty's response assessed and any catastrophic haemorrhage controlled, the next priority is to assess and ensure a clear and open airway.

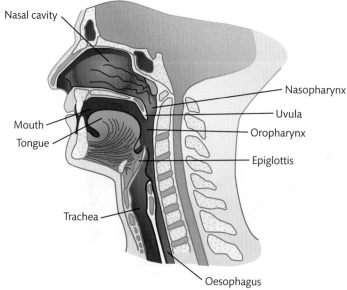

Figure 2.4 Anatomy of the upper airway

In order to breathe, a casualty requires a clear and open airway. Air is inhaled typically through the nostrils into the nasal cavity. The nostrils are separated by the septum – a thin dividing wall of bone and cartilage bone.

Air can also be introduced through the mouth into the oropharynx, the area at the back of the mouth below the nasopharynx. As most people breathe through their nose at rest, a casualty who is breathing through their mouth could be a cause for concern.

Also at the back of the mouth is the uvula, a soft fleshy protrusion that can be seen in an open mouth. The purpose of the uvula includes the production of saliva, speech and closing of the nasopharynx during swallowing.

Beyond the nasopharynx and oropharynx is the epiglottis. This cartilage flap separates the oesophagus (the food pipe) from the trachea (the wind pipe). In relaxed position the trachea is naturally open, only closing during swallowing as the epiglottis is pulled forwards to prevent food entering the lower airway.

Assessing the airway

For all unconscious casualties, inspect the mouth to ensure there is nothing in the airway; this could be fluids such as blood, vomit or mucus, or solids such as food, tablets or debris. If there is any blockage, it should be cleared immediately. If suction is immediately available, this should be used for fluids but it is usually more expedient to remove any obstruction with postural drainage. Pull the casualty towards you to allow fluids or solids to fall from the mouth; if necessary, a gloved finger can sweep the inside of the cheek. For an infant casualty, use only your little finger and with extreme caution; the mouth of an infant is both delicate and small.

> **Link**
>
> See page 85 for further information on airway management.

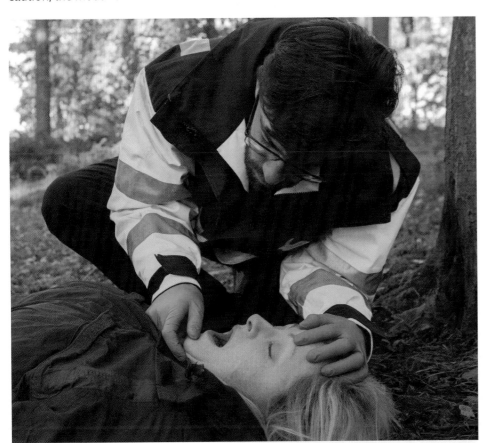

Check the airway for any obstructions

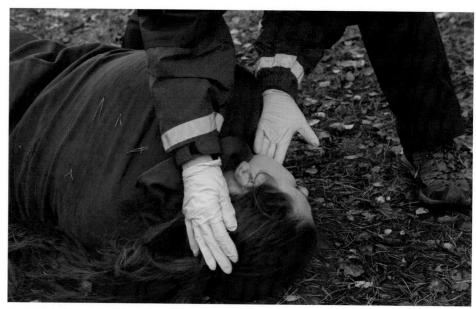

Postural drainage allows fluids to drain from the mouth

Quick tip

The finger sweep technique is the same for adults, children and infants.

Do not attempt to remove obstructions by inserting fingers into the mouth with the casualty on their back as:

▶ fluids cannot be removed in this way

▶ solids are likely to be pushed down further

▶ the casualty may bite you

▶ stimulating the back of the throat may stimulate the gag reflex, causing the casualty to vomit.

Opening the airway

Once you have ensured the airway is clear, open the airway.

If no spinal injury is suspected, open the casualty's airway by tilting the head backwards; the repositioning of the head will lift the tongue from the back of the casualty's airway.

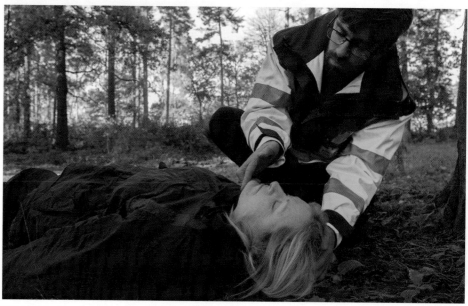

Tilt the head backwards to open the airway

Infants do not need their airway extended as much as adults, but, due to the disproportion of an infant's large head in comparison to its small torso, consider laying the infant either in your arms or with their torso on a thick blanket (but not under their head). This will allow the head to rest backwards keeping the airway open without excessive strain on the neck.

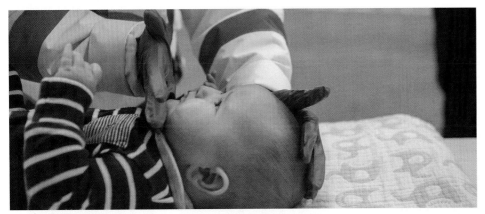

Link

See Unit 1, page 14, for more information on the mechanism of injury.

Link

See Opening the airway on page 86, for more information on jaw thrust.

Do not tilt an infant's head backwards as you would for an adult

If, based on the **mechanism of injury**, a spinal injury is suspected, the airway will need to be opened using the jaw thrust manoeuvre.

Explore the techniques used to manage choking casualties

Choking: adults

Choking is an airway issue that requires immediate intervention. The first action is to determine if the casualty is suffering from a complete airway obstruction or a partial airway obstruction.

▶ **Table 2.4**

Partial airway obstruction	Complete airway obstruction
• Breathing laboured, gasping or noisy • Some air escaping from the mouth • Casualty coughing or making a 'crowing' noise • Extreme anxiety or agitation • Pale or blueish skin colour	• Unable to effectively cough, breathe or speak, with no air movement • Casualty making obvious efforts to breathe with in-drawing of spaces between the ribs and above the collarbones • Face is greyish in colour with blue lips, due to lack of oxygen • Casualty is clutching the throat with both hands (the universal sign for choking)

Managing a partial airway obstruction

A partial obstruction should not need any physical intervention to clear but the anxious casualty who is panicking may require verbal instruction to focus on managing their own airway effectively.

▶ Ask the casualty 'Are you choking?' to determine whether their airway is completely blocked.

▶ If the casualty is able to verbalise a response, assume the casualty has a partial airway obstruction.

▶ Encourage the casualty to cough and expel the foreign body.

▶ Reassure and encourage the casualty.

▶ Stay with the casualty until full recovery has occurred.

Managing a complete airway obstruction

1 If the casualty is not able to respond to the question 'Are you choking?', assume the casualty has a complete airway obstruction.

2 Ask the casualty to cough.

3 If the casualty cannot cough, administer up to five back slaps.
   • With the casualty leaning forward, support the casualty's chest with one hand.
   • With the other hand, slap the casualty with the heel of the hand, on the back, high up, between the shoulder blades up to five times.
   • Check between each back slap to see if the obstruction has been cleared.

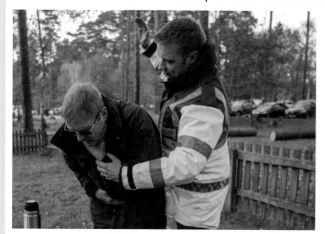
Adult back blows – body position

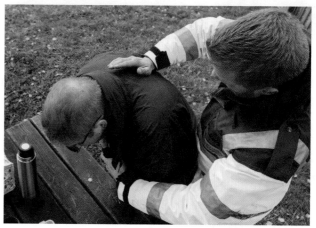
Adult back blows – aim for between the shoulder blades

4 If five back slaps do not clear the blockage, administer up to five abdominal thrusts.
   • Standing behind the casualty, place your arms around the casualty's abdomen.
   • Make a fist with one hand and place it between the casualty's umbilicus and xiphisternum.
   • Hold your clenched fist with the other hand.
   • Pull inward and upwards hard and fast.
   • Check between each abdominal thrust to see if the obstruction has cleared.

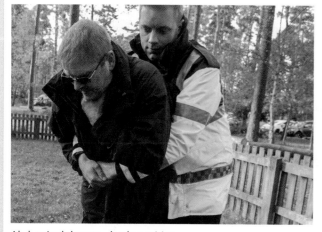
Abdominal thrusts – body position

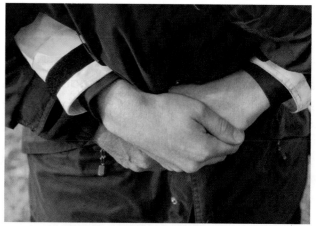
Abdominal thrusts – the clenched fist should be positioned in the centre of the abdomen

continued on page 53

Managing a complete airway obstruction (*continued*)

5 If abdominal thrusts do not clear the obstruction, alternate between up to five back slaps and up to five abdominal thrusts until the obstruction is cleared.

6 If the obstruction is not cleared and the casualty becomes unresponsive:
- support the casualty to the ground
- call the emergency services immediately
- begin CPR with chest compressions.

7 If chest compressions dislodge the blockage, the airway should be cleared immediately (see page 49 Assessing the airway).

8 If chest compressions or abdominal thrusts are performed to clear the blockage, refer the casualty to hospital for assessment as both procedures may cause abdominal or chest injury.

Choking: children and infants

The management of a choking child or infant differs to that of an adult because:

▶ the child or infant may not have the cognitive ability to interact with the responder as an adult would

▶ the physiology of a child or infant demands less aggressive intervention due to the risk of injury.

Recognising a choking child or infant

▶ The child or infant is either not breathing or has difficulty breathing.

▶ The onset of a breathing problem is sudden.

▶ There are no other associated illnesses.

▶ There is evidence around the casualty such as small toys or food.

To assess the severity of the situation and to determine if the airway obstruction is partial or complete, look for the casualty's ability to cough (and whether their cough is ineffective or effective).

▶ **Table 2.5**

Effective coughing: child/infant	Ineffective coughing: child/infant
• They are able to cry and make verbal responses to questions • They can cough loudly • They can take a breath before coughing • They are fully responsive	• They are unable to vocalise • They have quiet or silent coughs • They are unable to breathe • They have a blueish skin colour (cyanosis) • Their level of consciousness is decreasing

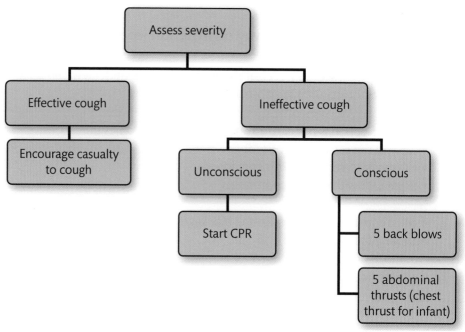

Figure 2.5 Effective and ineffective coughing

Effective coughing

▶ If the child is coughing effectively, then no external manoeuvre is necessary. Encourage the child to cough, and monitor continuously.

▶ If the child's coughing is, or is becoming, ineffective, shout for help immediately and determine the child's level of consciousness.

Ineffective coughing: child over 1 year   `3 Steps`

1 If the child is still conscious but has absent or ineffective coughing, give back blows.
  • Back blows are more effective if the child is positioned head-down.
  • A small child may be placed across the rescuer's lap, as with an infant.
  • If this is not possible, support the child in a forward-leaning position and deliver the back blows from behind.

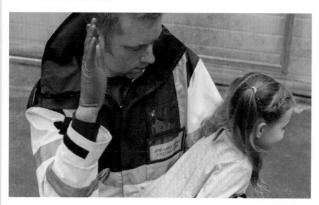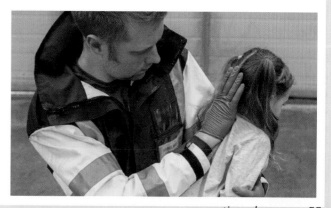

continued on page 55

Ineffective coughing: child over 1 year (*continued*)

2 If back blows do not relieve choking, give abdominal thrusts.
- Stand or kneel behind the child. Place your arms under the child's arms and encircle their torso.
- Clench your fist and place it between the umbilicus and xiphisternum.
- Grasp this hand with your other hand and pull sharply inwards and upwards.
- Repeat up to four more times.
- Ensure that pressure is not applied to the xiphoid process or the lower rib cage as this may cause abdominal trauma.
- The aim is to relieve the obstruction with each thrust rather than to give all five.

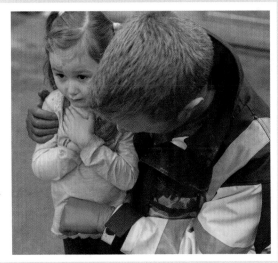

3 Following abdominal thrusts, reassess the child.
- If the object has not been expelled and the child is still conscious, continue the sequence of back blows and abdominal thrusts.
- Call out, or send, for help if it is still not available.
- Do not leave the child at this stage.
- If the object is expelled successfully, assess the child's clinical condition. It is possible that part of the object may remain in the respiratory tract and cause complications. If there is any doubt, summon medical assistance.

Ineffective coughing: infant
`3 Steps`

1 If the infant is still conscious but has absent or ineffective coughing, give back blows.
- Support the infant in a head-downwards, prone position, to enable gravity to assist removal of the foreign body.
- A seated or kneeling rescuer should be able to support the infant safely across their lap.
- Support the infant's head by placing the thumb of one hand at the angle of the lower jaw, and one or two fingers from the same hand at the same point on the other side of the jaw.
- Do not compress the soft tissues under the infant's jaw, as this will exacerbate the airway obstruction.
- Deliver up to five sharp back blows with the heel of one hand in the middle of the back between the shoulder blades.
- The aim is to relieve the obstruction with each blow rather than to give all five.

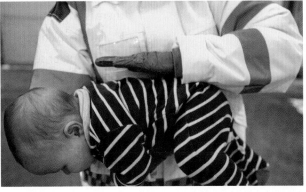

continued on page 56

Ineffective coughing: infant (*continued*)

2 If back blows fail to dislodge the object, and the infant is still conscious, use chest thrusts. Do not use abdominal thrusts for infants.

- Turn the infant into a head-downwards supine (lying down) position. This is achieved safely by placing your free arm along the infant's back, supporting the head.
- Support the infant down your arm, which is placed down (or across) your thigh.
- Identify the landmark for chest compression (approximately a finger's breadth above the xiphisternum – the lowest part of the sternum).
- Deliver up to five chest thrusts. These are similar to chest compressions, but sharper in nature and delivered at a slower rate.
- The aim is to relieve the obstruction with each thrust rather than to give all five.

3 Following chest thrusts, reassess the infant.

- If the object has not been expelled and the victim is still conscious, continue the sequence of back blows and chest thrusts.

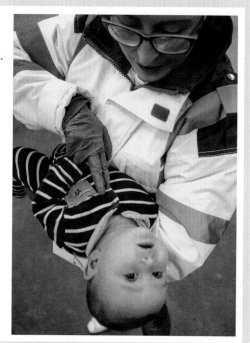

If the object is expelled successfully, assess the child's clinical condition. It is possible that part of the object may remain in the respiratory tract and cause complications. If there is any doubt, summon medical assistance.

▶ If the choking child is – or becomes – unconscious, place them on a firm, flat surface.

▶ Call out, or send, for help if it is still not available.

▶ Do not leave the child at this stage.

▶ Commence infant or child CPR.

Breathing

Anatomy of the lower airway

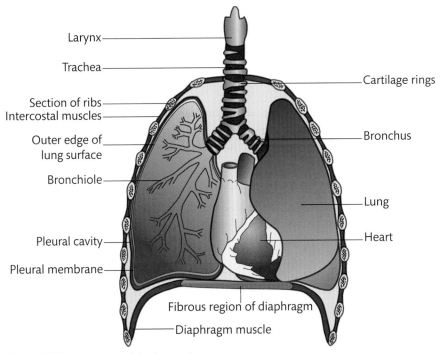

Figure 2.6 The anatomy of the lower airway

The trachea is the main conduit between the lungs and the upper airway. Just below the epiglottis is the larynx; commonly called the voice box. A casualty who has had a tracheostomy may have a stoma – a surgical opening made in their trachea, through their neck, to enable them to breathe.

The trachea separates into two bronchi and from there divides into smaller bronchioles within the lungs. Bronchioles will divide several times, each time becoming smaller, terminating in the alveoli – small air sacs and the site of gaseous exchange between oxygen, carbon dioxide and the blood.

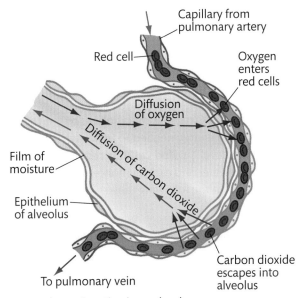

Figure 2.7 Gaseous exchange in action in an alveolus

Functions of the respiratory system

Ventilation, inspiration and expiration

Ventilation is the movement of air in and out of the lungs in order to supply the body with oxygen and remove carbon dioxide. Each ventilation comprises an inspiration phase and an expiration phase. Inhalation is achieved by two simultaneous actions:

1 contraction of the diaphragm (a bell shaped muscle below the lungs) that flattens downwards

2 contraction of the intercostal muscles that lifts the ribs upwards.

Both of these actions increase volume within the chest and subsequently reduce the pressure inside. Air (at a higher atmospheric pressure) outside the body moves in to fill this space until air pressure inside the lungs is equal to the air pressure outside.

As the diaphragm relaxes, moving back up into its original bell shape, and the intercostal muscles relax, causing the ribs to drop, the space within the chest is reduced, air pressure is increased and air is forced outwards.

Lung volumes and capacities

The volume of the air within the lung can be measured at different phases of ventilation.

▸ Table 2.6

Tidal volume (TV)	The amount of air inspired and expired during normal breathing, typically about 500 ml in a normal adult.
Inspiratory reserve volume (IRV)	The additional air that can be forcibly inhaled after the inspiration of a normal tidal volume – approximately 3100 ml.
Expiratory reserve volume (ERV)	The additional air that can be forcibly exhaled after the expiration of a normal tidal volume – approximately 1200 ml.
Residual volume (RV)	The volume of air still remaining in the lungs after the expiratory reserve volume is exhaled. This can only be calculated, not measured.
Total lung capacity (TLC)	The maximum amount of air that can fill the lungs (TLC = TV + IRV + ERV + RV) = approximately 6000 ml.
Vital capacity (VC)	The total amount of air that can be expired after fully inhaling (VC = TV + IRV + ERV = approximately 80% TLC). The value varies according to age and body size – approximately 4800 ml.

Gaseous exchange

Oxygen is a vital component for life. Oxygen is metabolised by the cells, along with glucose and fatty acids to produce energy needed to fulfil each cell's function. This metabolic process at the cellular level is called **cellular respiration**. The waste products of this process include water and carbon monoxide. The composition of inspired and expired air is shown in the following table.

▸ Table 2.7

Component	Inspired air	Expired air
Oxygen	≈ 21%	≈ 16%
Nitrogen	≈ 79%	≈ 79%
Carbon dioxide	≈ 0.04%	≈ 4%

Key term

Cellular respiration – metabolic processes that take place in the cells of organisms to convert biochemical energy from nutrients into adenosine triphosphate and then release waste products.

When fresh inspired air reaches the alveoli, the oxygen diffuses across the membrane into the surrounding capillaries, binding to red blood cells. Carbon dioxide, along with water as a waste product, is diffused across the membrane into the alveoli for expiration.

Assessment of breathing

Recognising **how** the casualty is breathing is as important as recognising if the casualty is breathing. Normal breathing is subtle and can be difficult to detect. In order to effectively assess breathing you are likely to need to be close to the casualty. For the unconscious casualty, place one ear close to the casualty's mouth and look down the body. In this position you can look at the chest rise and fall, listen for sounds of breathing and feel their breath on your cheek.

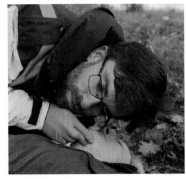
Checking for breathing

▶ **Table 2.8**

Characteristics	Normal	Abnormal
Rate	12–20 breaths per minute	Less than 10 and more than 30 breaths per minute are considered critical
Rhythm	Regular	Irregular, gasping, pauses
Depth	Normal	Ineffective shallow breaths Deep, heavy breaths
Effort	No effort	Visible effort
Noise	Silent	Gasping, wheezing, gurgling

Normal breathing should be quiet, regular and effortless. Any changes to a casualty's breathing are usually a symptomatic response to injury or illness. Notice how the casualty is breathing and record it.

If you have reason to suspect chest injury, based on the mechanism of injury or the nature of the breathing (e.g. blood in the airway), proceed to an exposed examination of the chest.

Physical examination for chest injury

To ensure your assessment of chest injury is both effective and standardised, the prompt RVP FLASH is used.

▶ **Table 2.9**

Rate	Record the rate of breaths per minute. This can be done over 15 seconds then doubling the number of recorded breaths and doubling again (or multiply by 4).
Volume	Is there enough volume of air being ventilated to be detectable easily? Is it noticeably too much? Does breathing appear an effort?
Put oxygen on now	Set up oxygen and administer in line with guidance.
Feel	With flat hands, completely surround the chest, feeling for an injury or deformity.
Look	Remove clothing and look at the skin for any signs of injury.
Armpits	Remember to check in the armpits and...
Sides	...that the chest includes the sides and the back
Holes	If there is an open chest wound, treat it now.

If any chest injury is found, it is treated now. You will learn about managing chest injuries in Unit 3.

Link

Information on how to deal with a casualty who is not breathing is found in the Principles of basic life support section of this unit on page 70.

Link

See Unit 1, page 14, for more information on the mechanism of injury.

Link

See the section on supplemental oxygen on page 94.

Link

See Unit 3, page 144, for more information on the management of chest injuries.

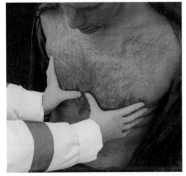
Fully expose the chest to complete an effective chest examination

Circulation

The heart is a muscular pump that forces blood around the body through a system of blood vessels – namely arteries, veins and capillaries. Together this is known as the cardiovascular system.

Blood is not a solution of components that are dissolved but a suspension of components that are carried in the plasma.

▶ **Table 2.10**

Plasma	A clear fluid that comprises approximately 55% of total blood volume. Plasma is important not only for carrying the other components but also for regulating blood pressure by shunting in or out of the cardiovascular system into intracellular spaces.
Red blood cells	Red blood cells account for approximately 45% of total blood volume. Their purpose is to transport oxygen molecules around the body.
White blood cells	White blood cells help fight infection.
Platelets	Platelets form clots to stop bleeding and heal wounds.

You can see that blood serves a number of functions beyond simply transporting oxygen. The cardiovascular system also has additional functions:

▶ removal of waste products of respiration (carbon dioxide and water)

▶ distribution of heat around the body through **vasodilation** and **vasoconstriction**

▶ transportation of hormones, nutrients, salts enzymes and urea

▶ fighting infections

▶ clotting.

Anatomy of the heart

The adult heart is the size of a closed fist, located in the thoracic cavity between the lungs and protected by the rib cage. It is surrounded by a tough membrane, the pericardium, which contains a thin film of fluid to prevent friction.

The heart is a double pump. Each side consists of a muscular upper chamber (the atria) and lower chamber (the ventricles). The right side of the heart pumps deoxygenated blood from the veins to the lungs for re-oxygenation. The left side of the heart pumps oxygenated blood from the lungs to the body.

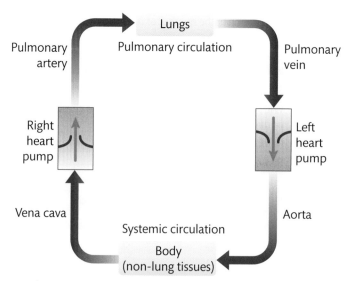

Figure 2.8 Diagram showing the double circulation of blood

Deoxygenated blood leaves the right ventricle via the pulmonary artery towards the lungs. Oxygenated blood returns to the left atrium from the lungs via the pulmonary veins.

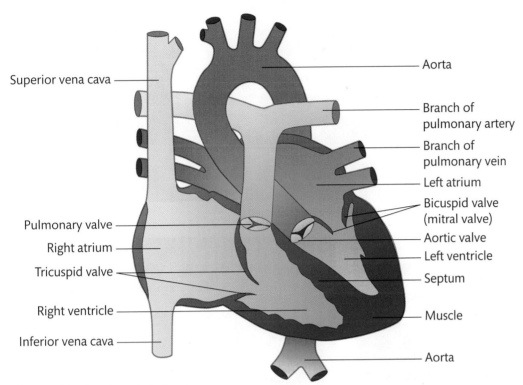

Superior vena cava

Pulmonary valve

Right atrium

Tricuspid valve

Right ventricle

Inferior vena cava

Aorta

Branch of pulmonary artery

Branch of pulmonary vein

Left atrium

Bicuspid valve (mitral valve)

Aortic valve

Left ventricle

Septum

Muscle

Aorta

Figure 2.9 Section through the heart

To ensure blood only flows in one direction through the heart there are a number of valves. Oxygenated blood in the left atrium is forced through the bicuspid valve into the left ventricle. From here it is forced through the aortic valve out of the heart through the aorta to supply the body with oxygen.

Returning deoxygenated blood enters the right atrium through the vena cava. The superior vena cava carries blood from the head and neck and the inferior vena cava carries blood from the rest of the body. From the right atrium blood is forced through the tricuspid valve into the right ventricle and again forced through the pulmonary valve into the pulmonary artery, and the cycle continues.

Assessing circulation

Checking a casualty's pulse is one way of assessing circulation but it is not the only method nor is it the most reliable.

Pulse

There are a number of places you can check for a pulse on a casualty; for an adult or child you may feel for a pulse at the neck (carotid artery) or at the wrist (radial artery). When looking for a pulse on an infant, there is too much fat around the neck and the structures are too delicate for us to apply pressure. The pulse at the wrist is likely to be too weak given the small size of their blood vessels. You may detect a pulse on the inside of the upper arm (brachial artery).

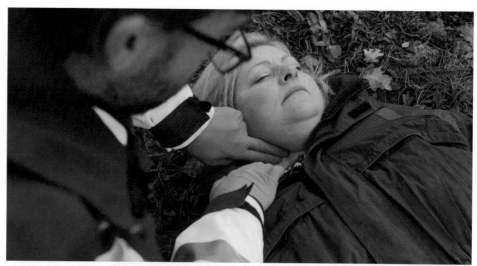

Checking the carotid pulse in an adult (or child)

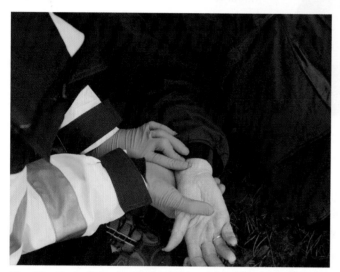

Checking the radial pulse in an adult (or child)

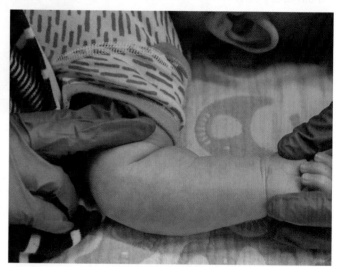

Checking the brachial pulse in an infant

A normal pulse in an adult should be regular and between 60 and 100 beats per minute; it is much faster in infants.

▶ **Table 2.11**

Age	Normal pulse rate (*beats per minute*)
12 years +	60–100
6–11 years	75–118
3–5 years	80–120
1–2 years	98–140
1 month–1 year	100–190
Less than 1 month	100–205

You may also notice the quality of the pulse; is it strong or weak? Is it regular or irregular?

There are, however, a number of problems with attempting to find a pulse:

▶ Skill decay – this is a practical skill that requires regular practise to ensure accuracy.

▶ You might be experiencing panic or stress.

▶ Extremely cold casualties will lose **peripheral circulation**.

▶ Casualties with low blood pressure will lose peripheral circulation.

▶ If your hands are cold, you may lose sensation.

Due to these issues you should also look for other signs of circulation.

Colour

▶ **Table 2.12**

Normal	A normal colour increases our confidence that the casualty has normal circulation.
Pale	This signifies a lack of blood at the skin. This could be because the casualty is cold and vasoconstriction at the skin is shunting warm blood to the core. It could be because the casualty is losing blood and the same vasoconstriction is shunting oxygenated blood to the core, or it might signify a lack of oxygen.
Blue (cyanosis)	If any of the problems above are not corrected, the casualty will begin to show a blue tinge. This happens peripherally first (peripheral cyanosis) at the fingers and toes but is more of a concern if the casualty is displaying a blue tinge at the face, and around the lips and eyes (central cyanosis).
Red	Heat, illness or other complications can cause blood to be pushed to the surface, showing as a redness in the casualty.
Yellow	A yellow tinge to the skin and eyes might indicate jaundice, for example.

Changes in skin colour are not always as noticeable on casualties with a strong ethnicity – higher concentrations of melanin (the pigment that determines skin normal skin colour) can mask the changes you see in Caucasian casualties.

▶ All skin colours will change but to various degrees – while you may not recognise a change in skin colour it may be because you do not know what 'normal' is for the casualty. Can anyone else around you verify the casualty's skin colour has changed?

▶ Other factors are linked to skin colour:
  • A pale casualty would feel cold.
  • A casualty with a red skin tone would feel warm.
  • Jaundice may not be visible.

Temperature

In addition to all other signs of circulation, a casualty whose skin is warm has enough blood in them. A cold casualty, in contrast, may have lost blood or may be hypothermic. A hot casualty may have a heat illness or infection.

Key term

Peripheral circulation – circulation at the extremities, i.e. the hands and feet.

Link

See Unit 1, page 9, for more information on skill decay.

Capillary refill

Pressing your thumb on the forehead of a casualty for a few seconds and then releasing will reveal a pale patch as you have pushed blood out of that area. Colour will normally resume within 2 seconds. This demonstrates the casualty has enough, circulating blood.

▶ If the casualty does not have enough blood, the forehead will be pale and the white patch will not be evident.

▶ If the casualty does not have circulating blood (or poor circulation) the white patch will remain for longer.

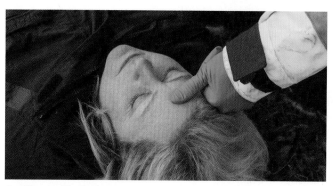

Capillary refill – before

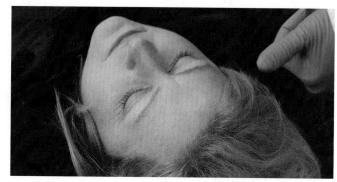

Capillary refill – after

Quick tip

Capillary refill does not work on casualties with dark skin; instead, apply the check on one of the casualty's finger nails. The finger nails are not affected by ethnicity but, being peripheral, the refill time is affected much more by the cold than when assessed at the forehead.

Link

See Unit 3, page 139, for more information on the management of bleeding.

Bleeding

With the exception of catastrophic bleeding, which will have been assessed and, if required, managed earlier on, you should now look for other bleeding.

It is important to note that bleeding may not always be obvious:

▶ Blood may pool underneath the casualty.

▶ Blood may soak into clothing, so the more clothing the casualty is wearing, the harder it is to find.

▶ Dark clothing will hide bleeding – blood simply looks wet in dark clothes.

▶ On dark tarmac, under orange street lights, blood will not be distinguishable from other fluids or water on the floor.

▶ Blood will soak into porous surfaces such as grass, gravel, sand or soil.

It is for all of these reasons that you must look thoroughly for bleeding. This should be carried out quickly and discreetly, however, as (for reasons of dignity and protection from the environment) you should not expose the casualty unnecessarily.

If the mechanism of injury suggests serious bleeding or multiple injuries, it may be judicious to cut away all clothing as a matter of course. The following photos show how to quickly expose a casualty by cutting clothing.

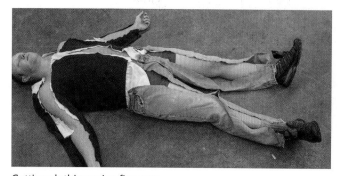

Cutting clothing using five cuts

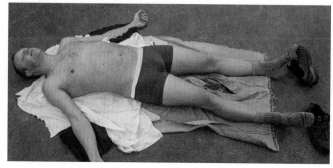

Exposed casualty

If the mechanism of injury does not suggest serious bleeding or multiple injury, you should check for serious bleeding by using the natural openings of the clothing: reaching into and around the collar, under jackets and jumpers, under the cuffs of sleeves and the hem of trousers. If blood is found, you need to access the source of the bleeding to apply direct pressure; this is most quickly achieved by cutting clothing rather than attempting to undress the casualty or reach under clothing.

Disability

After life-threating complications have been assessed and managed (airway problems, breathing problems and issues of circulation) you will now assess the casualty for disability of **nervous or endocrine systems**.

There are limitations in how much is achievable in a pre-hospital environment but you should consider the following.

Pupils

A useful mnemonic is PEARL: the casualty's **P**upils should be **E**qual **A**nd **R**eactive to **L**ight.

▶ If the casualty is unconscious, open the casualty's eye by placing light pressure on the upper rim of the eye socket, just below the eyebrow. Pull the skin upwards and the eyelid will follow. Do not press on the casualty's eye!

- On exposure to light the pupil should react by constricting (getting smaller). This is a subtle change that happens quickly.
- Afterwards check the other eye in the same manner; the same should happen.
- Both pupils should react to light and both should be the same size.

▶ If the casualty is conscious or their eyes are already open, notice the size of the pupils to begin with (they should be the same) and then shine a pen torch across one eye, and then the other, looking for a reaction.

This may identify a number of potential problems.

> **Quick check**
>
> What is a normal range for an adult pulse?

> **Key terms**
>
> **Nervous system** – the system comprising the brain, spinal cord and nerves.
>
> **Endocrine system** – relating to hormone production and regulation.

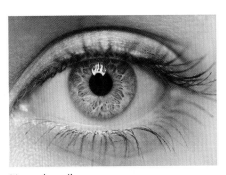

Normal pupil

▶ **Table 2.13**

Pupils	Possible cause
Dilated, unreactive	Cardiac arrest; certain drugs (LSD, Amphetamine); unconscious
Constricted, unreactive	CNS disease; certain drugs (Heroin, Morphine, Codeine)
Unequal	Stroke; head injury; pre-existing abnormality

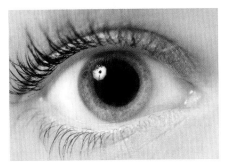

Dilated pupil

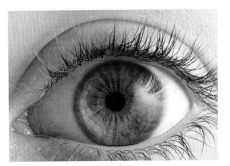

Constricted pupil

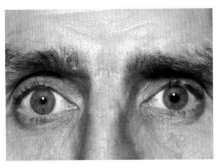

Unequal pupils

Colour sensation and movement (CSM)

CSM is another useful mnemonic to help in the assessment of the casualty; in this instance, it is for damage to underlying structures, namely blood vessels and nerves. Injuries (which you may have yet to find) will either cause damage to soft tissue (skin, muscle, fat), bones or joints, all of which are capable of healing relatively well if treated quickly and given the right care. Damage to blood vessels or nerves may cause more serious damage that is not as obvious as the original injury.

▶ Damage to blood vessels can deprive a body part or limb of oxygenated blood, causing potentially serious or life-threatening injuries.

▶ Damage to nerves can result in a loss of function. In addition, nerve damage is much harder, sometimes impossible, to repair.

Colour

Compare the colour of the limbs at the extremities (hands and feet) of the casualty. Compare each side to the other.

Sensation

If the casualty is conscious, ask them if they have any abnormal sensations such as numbness or **paraesthesia**. If the casualty is unconscious, attempt to administer a small amount of measured pain by pressing your thumb into the sole of each foot and the soft area between the thumb and the index finger. Is there a normal response to pain (e.g. withdrawing from the pain or a reaction shown in the face)? Is the response the same in each limb?

Movement

If the casualty is conscious, ask them to make a series of purposeful movements such as wiggling their toes or making a clenched fist. It is not possible to assess movement if the casualty is unconscious.

▶ A loss of colour, sensation or movement identified at the extremity in one limb would suggest damage to blood vessels or nerves at the point of injury.

▶ A loss of sensation or movement in a pair of limbs (e.g. both hands or both feet) or both limbs on one side might suggest nerve damage due to spinal cord injury or a problem with normal brain function.

Blood glucose

Blood glucose is regulated by the production of insulin in the pancreas, part of the endocrine system and the only function you can assess in this system. When you think of blood glucose, you think of diabetes and either *hypo* or *hyper* glycaemia, but it is important to remember that **everyone** is susceptible to low blood sugar.

Any casualty who is displaying a reduced level of consciousness or is behaving 'out of character' should be assessed for blood sugar levels using a glucometer (commonly called a 'blood glucose meter' or a 'glucose testing kit').

Expose

If you have not already done so, and if the mechanism of injury suggests it is necessary, the casualty should be exposed to assess injuries fully.

Factors to consider before removing all clothes include:

▶ **Is there a need?** If the issue is due to an illness, there is no need to remove clothing. If the issue is due to an injury, the removal of clothing may be required, but if the mechanism suggests a single injury, there may only be a need to expose the injured part of the body. If the mechanism suggests multiple, complex or life-threatening injuries, there may be a need to fully expose the casualty.

Key term

Paraesthesia – often called 'pins and needles', a usually temporary tingling, burning or pricking sensation, often in the arms or legs. It is caused by pressure on the nerves or the blood vessels that supply the nerves.

Link

For more on diabetes, see Unit 4, page 180.

Link

For more on the assessment and management of blood glucose, see Unit 4, page 182.

- **Environment:** in a cold environment fully exposing the casualty may be of more harm than the risk of not identifying an injury because the casualty is not exposed. Keep the casualty warm as being cold may compromise clotting capabilities.
- **Dignity:** if a casualty has a life-threatening injury, clothing is exposed but if the injuries are not life threatening, there is no need to expose someone beyond necessity in a crowded or populated environment.

The secondary survey

Response, Airway, Breathing, Circulation and Disability are often referred to as the primary survey – the initial assessment of immediately life-threatening injuries or conditions. Within Expose you will look for further evidence of injury or medical conditions. This is often referred to as the secondary survey.

The secondary survey follows a structured systematic approach:

- Always assess the casualty from head-to-toe to avoid being distracted by obvious injuries that may not be the most serious.
- Talk your way through the procedure – even if the casualty is unconscious, they may still hear what is going on around them.
- Look at the casualty's face for a response to pain throughout the assessment.

Do not treat injuries as you find them – the first injury you find may not be the only injury or the most serious. Instead, complete the full survey before deciding which injury warrants management first.

> **Table 2.14**

Head and neck	Check skull and jaw, cervical spine, ears, eyes, mouth, nose, and face. Note odours, blood or other fluids.
Shoulders	Compare both clavicles for symmetry. Press on the shoulders and notice any **crepitus** of bones or joints.
Chest	Check the sternum: place your fingers in a straight line along the sternum, press down and move your fingers up and down the sternum. The sternum is a lumpy, uneven bone but it is rigid. Note any crepitus. Check the ribs, with both hands flat on the chest. The ribs should feel smooth and continuous.
Abdomen	Divide the abdomen into four quadrants through the navel – press on each quadrant; each quadrant should feel the same with no swelling or rigidity that might indicate internal bleeding.
Lower spine	Examine without moving the casualty. Feel underneath the casualty for normal spinal alignment.
Pelvis	Do not press on the pelvis. Your suspicion of a pelvic injury is based solely on the mechanism of injury, given that it requires a large force to break the pelvis. If the pelvis is broken, pressing on the pelvis can cause further damage to underlying structures such as blood vessels or nerves. If you suspect a spinal injury, also suspect a pelvic injury. If you do not suspect a spinal injury, do not suspect a pelvic injury either.
Legs and arms	Examine in pairs, all the way around the limbs.
Pockets and personal effects	Empty all pockets – this may provide evidence of medical conditions (such as medication or medical information cards), may identify the casualty and will remove any objects that are likely to cause injury if the casualty is rolled onto them, such as coins and keys.

Key term

Crepitus – the sound and/or feeling of grating, usually associated with a fracture.

Continuing casualty assessment

After the primary and secondary survey have been completed, you are now in a period of evaluation of the casualty's vital signs including:

▶ level of response (which you may already have established)

▶ respirations

▶ pulse

▶ colour

▶ temperature

▶ capillary refill

▶ pupil size.

The first set of observations you have collected will serve as your benchmark. On their own they can give an indication of the casualty's state of health. When compared to ongoing observations over a period of time, they may show trends that might indicate an improvement or deterioration in the casualty's state of health, or if the casualty's vital signs are stable.

The conscious casualty

The DRCA(c)BCDE protocol works well when applied in the systematic method explained earlier but does not fit appropriately when applied to a conscious casualty with a minor injury or illness. It would not be appropriate to attempt a secondary assessment on a casualty whose only symptom is a headache, or to check the airway of a casualty who is telling you they feel fine, for example.

When managing a conscious casualty, you will still observe their vital signs but in a more subtle manner. What you can also gain from a conscious casualty is information.

Questioning the conscious casualty

The mnemonic SAMPLE is a prompt for pertinent questions that may help you diagnose the casualty's main complaint or discover underlying problems.

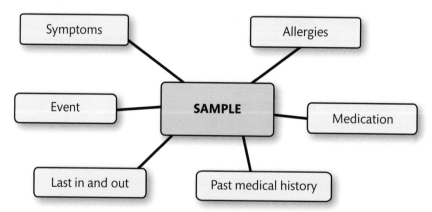

Figure 2.10 Which questions should you ask the casualty? Use the mnemonic SAMPLE to help you.

Symptoms

A sign is something you can see (bruising, swelling, bleeding for example) and you might find these on any casualty if you look properly. The symptoms are how the casualty feels. Only a conscious casualty can tell us their symptoms.

Symptoms include (but are not limited to):

▶ pain

▶ nausea

▶ headache

▶ dizziness

▶ heat/cold

▶ tiredness

▶ irritability.

None of these are visible, so you will need to ask the casualty. This may sound obvious but if the casualty has an injury, it is easy to become distracted by that injury. They are in pain, but how else do they feel?

Allergies

Does the casualty have any allergies? The problem may have been triggered by an allergy. It is also worth knowing what allergies they have medication for and this information will need to be communicated to other healthcare providers responsible for the casualty's treatment.

Medication

What medication is the casualty taking or has recently taken? You may be familiar with common medicines and you may even know what they are for, such as:

▶ Salbutamol (used in asthma inhalers)

▶ Insulin (a hormone controlling blood glucose levels)

▶ GTN (used to treat angina)

▶ Warfarin (a medicine that stops blood clotting).

If you are not familiar with the casualty's medications, ask further questions, such as:

▶ Do you need it now?

▶ Do you have it with you?

▶ When did you last take it?

Past medical history

You need to ask the casualty about any relevant past medical history, for example 'Has this happened before?'

With injuries you might ask: 'Is this a recurring problem or is this a new event?'; 'Have you had any surgery in that area?'

With illnesses: 'Is this something you have had before?'; 'Do you have any medication for it?'; 'Could your illness be related?'

Last in and out

When did the casualty last eat or drink? What was it? These may be clues to the casualty's condition. It is sometimes worth asking when they last went to the toilet.

Events

What happened? This alone can help you build up a bigger picture. Ideally get this information from the casualty if they are able to answer your questions. If not, ask bystanders what happened, but be aware: bystanders have a tendency to embellish, so listen to what they are saying, look at the scene around the casualty and look at the casualty to build up a representative picture.

SAMPLE is only a prompt; you do not have to ask these questions in this order and you do not necessarily need to use these terms. Many people will not know what a symptom is, so a better question might be 'How do you feel?' for example.

By asking the conscious casualty questions you will not just gather information, you will also be able to notice many of their vital signs. It is not simply what they say, but how they say it.

▶ **Table 2.15**

Response	Is the casualty speaking clearly and are their answers making sense?
Airway	If the casualty is speaking to you clearly and without effort, you can be certain the casualty has a clear and open airway.
Breathing	The casualty's speech will mirror their breathing; if their breathing is fast and weak, their speech is likely to be fast and quiet. If their breathing is slow and deep, their speech is likely to be slow and deep with pauses.

Quick tip

Never tell a casualty you are going to check their breathing because once they are aware of their breathing, it will change!

Assessment practice 2.1 (C, EC) 1.1

You are called late at night to a casualty who you find staggering outside a pub. You call to them and they turn around to look at you. They say something but you are not able to understand their slurred words.

1 How would you describe their level of response?

2 Explain how you have reached this conclusion.

3 What would be your initial actions to manage this casualty?

Assessment practice 2.2 (C, EC) 1.1, 6.1, 6.2, 6.3

A young male casualty is found conscious and fully alert in a workshop. He has cut his wrist on a piece of cutting equipment. Bystanders are applying direct pressure to the arterial bleed but it is not stopping the bleeding.

1 What would be your initial actions to manage this casualty?

2 Explain what is meant by the term 'catastrophic haemorrhage'?

3 Describe the process you would use to attempt to stop this bleed.

Assessment practice 2.3 (C, EC) 1.1, 3.1, 3.4, 3.7

You are in a restaurant when a parent starts frantically calling that their baby is not breathing.

1 What would be your initial actions to manage this casualty?

2 Explain how the management of a choking infant differs from that of a choking adult.

Explore the principles of basic life support for adults, children and infants

Basic life support is a key skill for any first aider or healthcare provider. Any casualty who is found not breathing, or not breathing normally, requires immediate treatment.

Principles of basic life support

For a casualty who is not breathing, the single most important factor in a successful resuscitation is timely defibrillation. The Chain of Survival describes four key stages that must be administered promptly and in sequence to ensure the prompt arrival and application of a defibrillator and the management of the casualty in the interim.

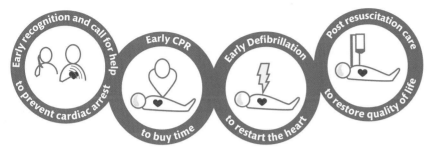

Figure 2.11 The four stages of the Chain of Survival

▶ **Early recognition and call for help**
Once the casualty has been determined as not breathing, the assumption is made that they are in **cardiac arrest**. Early recognition is critical to enable rapid activation of the ambulance service and prompt initiation of CPR.

▶ **Early CPR**
The immediate initiation of **cardiopulmonary resuscitation (CPR)** can double or quadruple the probability of survival from out-of-hospital cardiac arrest by maintaining some level of oxygenation to the brain.

▶ **Early defibrillation**
Defibrillation within 3–5 minutes of collapse can produce survival rates as high as 50–70 per cent. Each minute of delay to defibrillation reduces the probability of survival to hospital discharge by 10 per cent.

▶ **Early advanced life support and standardised post-resuscitation care**
Early defibrillation with prompt CPR may result in a successful pre-hospital resuscitation but the casualty will still need advanced treatment, drugs and assessment to ensure full recovery.

> **Key terms**
>
> **Cardiac arrest** – the cessation of blood circulating around the body.
>
> **Cardiopulmonary resuscitation (CPR)** – the dual action of oxygenating the blood and pumping the heart to maintain circulation of oxygenated blood to the brain.

Summoning assistance

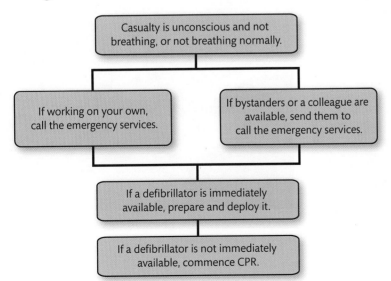

Figure 2.12 Summoning assistance and starting CPR promptly will help the casualty's chance of survival

Agonal breathing

Notice that the emergency services are also called and CPR is also anticipated for any casualty who is unconscious and **not breathing normally**. Any unconscious casualty found not breathing is also assumed to be in cardiac arrest.

Agonal breaths are irregular, slow and deep breaths, frequently accompanied by a characteristic snoring sound. They originate from the brain stem, which remains functioning for some minutes even when deprived of oxygen. This is often misinterpreted as the casualty breathing and that therefore CPR is not needed. Agonal breathing may be present in up to 40 per cent of casualties within the first five minutes of cardiac arrest.

Cardiopulmonary resuscitation (CPR)

Link

For more on supplemental oxygen, see page 94 of this unit.

The cardio element of CPR attempts to manually circulate the blood to maintain oxygenation of the brain. The pulmonary element of CPR oxygenates the blood from either the surrounding air, the rescuer's breath or with supplemental oxygen.

Chest compressions

▶ Kneeling beside the casualty, interlink the hands as shown in the following photos and place the heel of the lower hand directly on the centre of the chest.

▶ Lean up and over the casualty so your arms, locked straight at the elbow, are vertical. Your shoulders should be directly above your wrists.

▶ Commence chest compressions by compressing the chest 5–6 cm, 30 times at a rate of 100–120 compressions a minute (up to two compressions a second). If the casualty is not on a firm surface, move the casualty to the floor, otherwise adequate compression depth may be difficult to achieve.

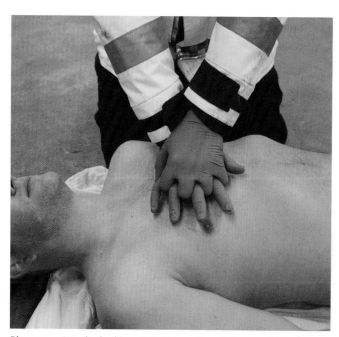

Place your interlocked hands in the centre of the casualty's chest

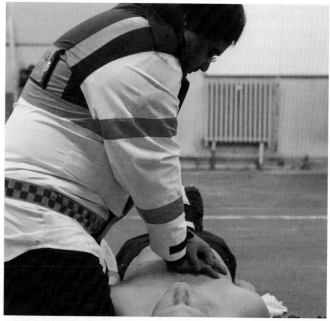

Position yourself so that your arms are perpendicular, shoulders directly above your hands

Rescue breaths – mouth-to-mouth

To oxygenate the casualty, the airway must be clear and open.

▸ Tilt the head back and pinch the nostrils closed to ensure no air escapes.

▸ Making a good seal around the casualty's mouth with yours, breathe into the casualty for one second; you are aiming to make the chest rise. (A normal breath is sufficient. Blowing into the casualty too hard, too fast or too much can cause air to inflate the stomach, resulting in vomit entering the casualty's airway and your mouth.)

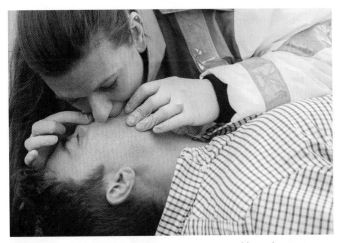

Allow the chest to deflate before giving a second breath

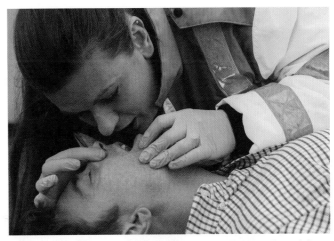

Do not interrupt compressions by more than 10 seconds to deliver two breaths

Variations on rescue breaths

Mouth-to-nose

If you are not able to make an effective seal with the casualty's mouth, due to facial injury, for example, or if there is obvious blood, vomit or other fluid evident on the casualty's lip that presents a risk of infection, it is possible to provide rescue breaths through the casualty's nose.

With the head tilted as before, and with one hand supporting the casualty's head, cover the casualty's mouth with the other hand. Make a good seal around the casualty's nostrils and breathe gently for one second as before, with the aim of getting the casualty's chest to rise.

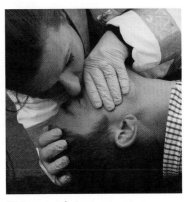

Giving mouth-to-nose rescue breaths

Pocket mask

The pocket mask is a small plastic mask that effectively seals the mouth and nose of the casualty and acts as a barrier between the casualty and the rescuer, preventing direct contact and reducing the risk of infection.

To use a pocket mask effectively, CPR is delivered at the casualty's head; chest compressions are delivered in the same manner, in the centre of the chest, by leaning forward over the casualty's head.

To deliver rescue breaths, the pocket mask is held onto the casualty's face with both hands, while the head is tilted back, opening the casualty's airway. With the pocket mask in position, place the heel of the thumbs on each side of the mask and your fingers behind the casualty's jaw. Squeeze the mask onto the casualty's face.

The temptation is to press down on the mask to create a seal but this risks closing the casualty's airway.

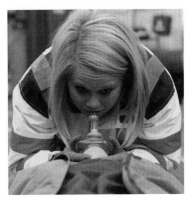

Pocket mask technique

Bag-valve mask

The bag-valve mask (BVM) comprises a pocket mask with a squeezable bag connected. This allows air from the atmosphere (at 21 per cent oxygen) to be forced into the casualty's lungs rather than from the rescuer's breath (at 16 per cent oxygen).

The use of a BVM also reduces the risk of infection as it does not require any direct contact with the casualty or allow for transition of breath or body fluids.

Single person technique

Kneeling beside the casualty, with their airway open, align the mask to the casualty's face. Hold the mask between your thumb and index finger and hook your little finger behind the angle of the jaw to bring the mask down onto the face to ensure a good seal. The other hand squeezes the bag.

The single person technique can be difficult and requires practice. Often it is a challenge to ensure a good seal with one hand (the most likely gap will be at the bridge of the nose where air will escape). Delivering a controlled ventilation can also be difficult with one hand especially if the responder's hands are small.

Each ventilation is delivered with the same aim: to see a rise and fall of the chest. Avoid overly vigorous ventilations as this risks inflating the stomach, which can lead to vomit entering the casualty's airway.

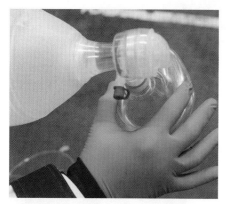
Hold the mask between your thumb and index finger

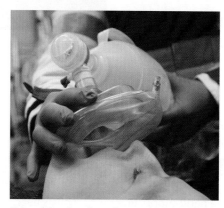
Using this grip, place the mask in position

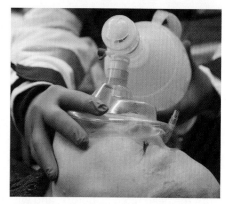
Hook your little finger behind the angle of the casualty's jaw

Two-person technique

Using a BVM with two people is easier and can be operated with greater control.

The assistant kneels at the head of the casualty and grips the mask with the heel of the thumb of each hand on each side of the mask. The assistant simultaneously maintains an open airway by tilting the head back while holding the mask to the casualty's face. A much more effective seal is made with two hands. Again, ensure your assistant avoids pushing down on the mask to create a seal as this risks closing the casualty's airway. Instead, squeeze the mask in place with your fingers behind the casualty's jaw.

Holding the mask in place is the sole responsibility of your assistant. The assistant can keep the BVM in place constantly or they can remove the BVM during compressions. If the BVM is removed during compressions, give your assistant a cue to replace the mask by counting down your last few compressions '26, 27, 28, 29, 30' so that the mask is in place, the seal is made and the casualty's airway is open, ready for you to deliver two ventilations.

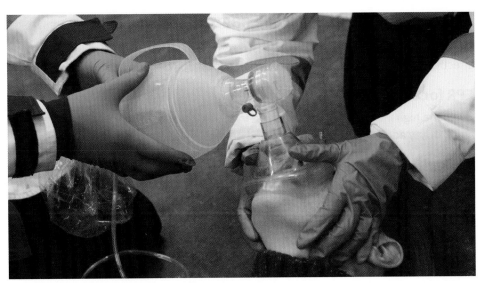
Bag-valve mask using a two-person technique

Both the pocket mask and BVM can be connected to supplemental oxygen.

Compression-only CPR

Since 2010 there has been global consensus that if the responder is either unwilling or unable to perform mouth-to-mouth or mouth-to-nose rescue breaths, continual chest compressions should be given instead.

Performing CPR can be psychologically challenging; one of the most difficult aspects for many people, especially members of the public, is the direct contact with the casualty's mouth and it is for this reason that many casualties who collapse do not receive CPR until a healthcare professional arrives.

If the responder is unwilling or unable to perform conventional CPR (thus depriving the brain of oxygen), rather than doing nothing, continual chest compressions should be encouraged. The main reason for delivering chest compressions is to pump blood manually around the body by squashing the heart between the sternum and the spine. This action will also mechanically ventilate the casualty, albeit to a lesser degree than mouth-to-mouth ventilations, by squashing air out of the chest with each compression and drawing air in each time the compression is released as the rib cage rebounds. An additional benefit to compression-only CPR is that each time compressions are stopped to provide the rescue breaths, the casualty's blood pressure drops, resulting in lower **perfusion** to the brain. It takes time to increase the blood pressure back up to the point at which blood will begin to circulate with compressions. If continual compressions are delivered, there may be less oxygen being ventilated but circulation and oxygen perfusion is continuous. Compression-only CPR will only be effective for the first few minutes.

Cessation of CPR

Continue CPR until:

▶ a health professional tells you to stop

▶ you become exhausted

▶ the casualty is definitely waking up, moving, opening eyes and breathing normally.

Turn the casualty to the safe airway position (also known as the recovery position) if they start breathing effectively but remain unconscious.

Key term

Perfusion – to supply with blood.

Link

See page 87 for more information on the safe airway position.

Modifications for special casualties

The guidance given earlier is for adult casualties. The method of delivering safe and effective CPR for some casualties is different depending on their age and physiology.

CPR for children

Given the high incidence of cardiac arrest in adults it is appropriate to assume cardiac arrest in any adult who is unconscious and not breathing or not breathing normally. Cardiac arrest in children and infants is less common than in adults. Children and infants are likely to go into **respiratory arrest**. CPR is unlikely to ever restart the heart (hence the onus on immediately summoning the emergency services and a defibrillator for adults). CPR is much more likely to restart breathing. For this reason, if a child or infant is found to be unconscious and not breathing or not breathing normally, the focus must be on resuscitation first and then summoning help.

The first action is to provide five rescue breaths.

Rescue breaths for an infant
`5 Steps`

1. Ensure a neutral position of the head (as an infant's head is usually flexed when supine, this may require some extension) and apply chin lift without placing your fingers under the chin bone.

2. Take a breath and cover the mouth and nasal apertures of the infant with your mouth, making sure you have a good seal. If the nose and mouth cannot both be covered in the older infant, the rescuer may attempt to seal only the infant's nose or mouth with his mouth (if the nose is used, close the lips to prevent air escape).

3. Blow steadily into the infant's mouth and nose over one second, sufficient to make the chest rise visibly. This is the same time period as in adult practice.

4. Maintaining the head position and chin lift, take your mouth away and watch for the chest to fall as air comes out.

5. Take another breath and repeat this sequence four more times.

Rescue breaths for a child over 1 year
`7 Steps`

1. Ensure the child's head is tilted and chin lifted.

2. Pinch the soft part of the nose closed with the index finger and thumb of your hand on the forehead.

3. Open the child's mouth a little, but maintain the chin lift.

4. Take a breath and place your lips around the child's mouth, making sure that you have a good seal.

5. Blow steadily into the mouth over one second, sufficient to make the chest rise visibly.

continued on page 77

Rescue breaths for a child over 1 year (*continued*)

6 Maintaining head tilt and chin lift, take your mouth away and watch for the child's chest to fall as air comes out.

7 Take another breath and repeat this sequence four more times. Identify effectiveness by seeing that the child's chest has risen and fallen in a similar fashion to the movement produced by a normal breath.

Check for signs of life   `5 Steps`

1 Take no more than 10 seconds to look for signs of life including any movement, coughing or normal breathing (not abnormal gasps or infrequent, irregular breaths).

2 If you check the pulse, take no more than 10 seconds.
- In a child aged over 1 year, feel for the carotid pulse in the neck.
- In an infant, feel for the brachial pulse on the inner aspect of the upper arm.

3 If confident that you can detect signs of circulation within 10 seconds, continue rescue breathing if necessary, until the child starts breathing effectively on their own.

4 Turn the child onto their side into the safe airway position if they start breathing effectively but remain unconscious. Continue compressions and breaths in a ratio of 15:2.

5 If there are no signs of life within 10 seconds, start chest compressions.

Chest compressions on an infant   `7 Steps`

1 To avoid compressing the upper abdomen, locate the xiphisternum by finding the angle where the lowest ribs join in the middle. Compress the sternum one finger's breadth above this.

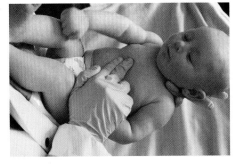

2 A first responder working alone should compress the sternum with the tips of two fingers.

3 Compression should be sufficient to depress the sternum by at least one third of the depth of the chest; the compression will be approximately 4 cm for an infant.

4 Release the pressure completely, then repeat at a rate of 100–120 min^{-1}.

continued on page 78

Chest compressions on an infant (*continued*)

5 Allow the chest to return to its resting position before starting the next compression.

6 After 15 compressions, tilt the head, lift the chin and give two effective breaths.

7 Continue compressions and breaths in a ratio of 15 : 2.

Encircling technique

3 Steps

If there are two or more rescuers, use the encircling technique.

1 Place both thumbs flat, side-by-side, on the lower half of the sternum (as earlier), with the tips pointing towards the infant's head.

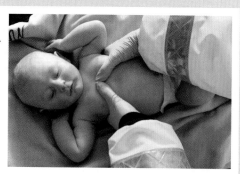

2 Spread the rest of both hands, with the fingers together, to encircle the lower part of the infant's rib cage with the tips of the fingers supporting the infant's back.

3 Press down on the lower sternum with your two thumbs to depress it at least one third of the depth of the infant's chest, approximately 4 cm.

Chest compressions on a child over 1 year

4 Steps

1 Place the heel of one hand over the lower half of the sternum (as earlier).

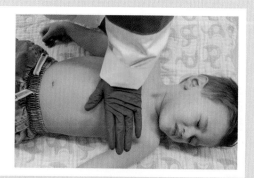

2 Lift the fingers to ensure that pressure is not applied over the child's ribs.

continued on page 79

Chest compressions on a child over 1 year (*continued*)

3 Position yourself vertically above the casualty's chest and, with your arm straight, compress the sternum to depress it by at least one-third of the depth of the chest; the compression will be approximately 5 cm.

4 In larger children, or for small rescuers, chest compressions may be achieved most easily by using both hands with the fingers interlocked. Continue compressions and breaths in a ratio of 15 : 2.

Summoning assistance
`3 Steps`

1 When more than one rescuer is available, one (or more) starts resuscitation while another summons assistance.

2 If only one rescuer is present, undertake resuscitation for about 1 minute before summoning assistance. To minimise interruptions in CPR, it may be possible to carry an infant or small child while summoning help.

3 Continue CPR until:
- the child shows signs of life (normal breathing, coughing, movement or definite pulse of greater than 60 per minute)
- further qualified help arrives
- you become exhausted.

Modifications to pregnant casualties

Cardiac arrest in pregnancy is rare. However, if it is suspected, normal adult protocols are applied with slight modifications to account for the changes in physiology of the pregnant casualty.

1 Hand position on the sternum may need to be 2–3 cm higher in the later stages (28 weeks+) of pregnancy.
2 Manually displace the uterus to the left to minimise compression of the vena cava by the fetus.
3 If it is possible, tilt the casualty to their left on a firm surface. This can be difficult to achieve as a soft surface, or packaging under the casualty, can often collapse under the weight of the casualty or may reduce the effectiveness of compressions.

Modifications to neck breathers

Some casualties may breathe through a stoma – a surgically implanted conduit through the neck into the trachea to enable them to breathe. A full neck breather will breathe exclusively through the stoma; the mouth and nose are completely disconnected from the trachea above the stoma, which may mean the casualty is unable to speak. A partial neck breather will still have a connection between the trachea and mouth and nose to enable speech and will usually have a plastic tube (tracheostomy tube) fitted with the stoma to keep it open.

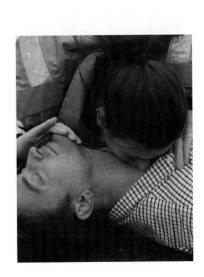

1 To perform rescue breaths, the head must be tilted back to open the airway.
2 If the casualty is a partial neck breather, use one hand to cover the mouth and pinch the nostrils to prevent air escaping. This is not necessary on a full neck breather.

3 Make a good seal around the stoma or the tracheostomy tube with your mouth.

4 Blow into the stoma, as usual, for one second to enable the chest to rise.

5 Allow air to escape before delivering the next breath.

6 It is sometimes possible to use an infant or child pocket mask or BVM over the stoma.

7 A BVM can be connected directly to the tracheostomy tube.

Link

See page 60 for the anatomy of the heart.

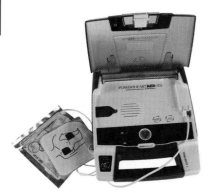

Defibrillator and pads

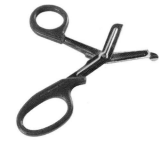

Scissors

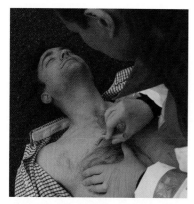

You may need to shave the casualty's chest

Defibrillation

The coordination of this sequence of the heart described earlier in this unit is controlled by the heart's own pacemaker – the Sino-Atrial Node (SA Node). This sends a signal across the atrium to the Atrio-Ventricular Node (AV Node), forcing the muscles to contract and pump blood into the ventricles. From here the signal passes down the Bundle Branches and around the Purkinje Fibres, which forces the ventricles to contract and pump blood away from the heart. The electrical activity is repolarised and the sequence begins again.

When the casualty is in cardiac arrest, there may be an electrical disturbance creating uncoordinated contractions (Ventricular Fibrillation) or contracting too quickly (Ventricular Tachycardia) to effectively pump blood. An Automated External Defibrillator (AED) may be able to depolarise the heart, stopping it momentarily to allow the SA Node to restart the contractions in a normal, coordinated manner.

When the AED electrodes are applied, the AED will analyse the rhythm of the heart; both Ventricular Fibrillation and Ventricular Tachycardia are considered 'shockable rhythms'. The AED is able to deliver a shock in these instances. If the casualty is not in cardiac arrest and has a normal heart rhythm or if there is no electrical activity at all (asystole) or the heart is in any other rhythm, the AED will not be able to deliver a shock.

The ability of the equipment to analyse the rhythm of the heart allows the rescuer to confidently apply an AED to the casualty without fear that the unconscious casualty who has incorrectly been diagnosed as not breathing will be shocked.

Equipment checks

Before the defibrillator is applied, and as part of your regular equipment checks, ensure the defibrillator and its components are in a satisfactory condition.

▶ **Table 2.16**

Item	Checks
Defibrillator	The defibrillator should be clean with no signs of damage. The defibrillator will have a visual cue to the battery level, typically a digital display or coloured LEDs.
Electrodes	The AED electrodes (or pads) must be unopened and in date.
Scissors	AED electrodes must be applied directly to the skin; a shirt can easily be ripped open but T-shirts, jumpers and underwear should be cut away for expediency.
Razor	If the casualty has a hairy chest, it is necessary to shave the chest; for this the AED should contain a razor.
Towel	The casualty's skin will need to be clean and dry before the electrode pads are applied; for this reason, it is sensible for the AED to contain a small towel.

Precautions and preparations

It is best practice when using supplemental oxygen to remove the non-rebreather mask or BVM and place one metre away – do not allow this to delay the delivery of a shock.

Ensure the casualty's chest is clean, dry and suitably exposed to allow correct placement of the pads.

The following table discusses some of the factors that can inhibit the correct placement or adhesion of the pads.

▶ **Table 2.17**

Problem	Solution
Sweat	Sweat or moisture on the skin will need to be dried to allow the pads to adhere.
Chest hair	Excessive chest hair will need to be shaved for the same reason. A disposable razor is often supplied with the AED for this purpose. Only the upper right portion of the chest needs to be shaved. Do not delay defibrillation if a razor is not immediately available.
Lotions	Sun lotions, insect repellent, moisturiser or other contaminants will need to be wiped from the skin.
Jewellery	You do not need to remove necklaces or piercings – this causes unnecessary delay – but do not place pads directly over them.
Medical patches	Transdermal patches such as nicotine or GTN patches are often foil backed. If an AED electrode is placed over a foil-backed patch, this will interfere with correct analysis of the heart rhythm. Remove patches.
Underwear	Bras interfere with correct pad placement; the right shoulder strap will interfere with correct placement of the upper right electrode and the chest strap will interfere with correct placement of the lower left electrode. The quickest and simplest way to remove the bra is to cut through it between each cup and expose the breast.

Poor pad contact can reduce the ability of the AED to accurately detect a rhythm. Most AEDs will verbally prompt the operator to re-apply the pads if pads are incorrectly placed or there is poor contact.

Correct pad placement

Although most AED electrodes carry a picture on them of correct pad placement, it does not matter if their positions are reversed – it is the position that is important, not the polarity. If you make a mistake, do not waste time removing the pads and re-placing them as they may not adhere correctly again when re-attached. Avoid placing the upper right pad too low and the lower left pad too frontal (the latter should be on the side of the chest).

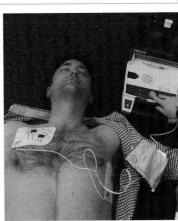

Correctly placed pads

Children and AEDs

Standard AED pads are suitable for use in children older than 8 years. Special paediatric pads, which attenuate the current delivered during defibrillation, should be used in children aged between 1 and 8 years old if they are available; if not, standard adult-sized pads should be used. The use of an AED is not recommended in children aged less than 1 year old. However, if an AED is the only defibrillator available its use should be considered (preferably with the paediatric pads described earlier).

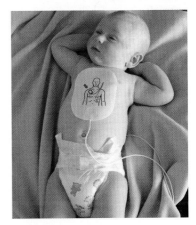

Pad placement on an infant

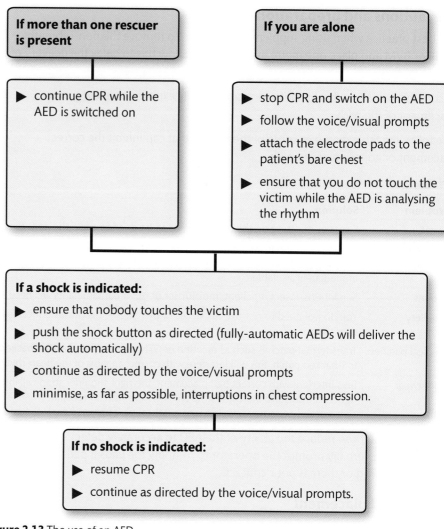

If more than one rescuer is present	If you are alone
▶ continue CPR while the AED is switched on	▶ stop CPR and switch on the AED ▶ follow the voice/visual prompts ▶ attach the electrode pads to the patient's bare chest ▶ ensure that you do not touch the victim while the AED is analysing the rhythm

If a shock is indicated:

▶ ensure that nobody touches the victim

▶ push the shock button as directed (fully-automatic AEDs will deliver the shock automatically)

▶ continue as directed by the voice/visual prompts

▶ minimise, as far as possible, interruptions in chest compression.

If no shock is indicated:

▶ resume CPR

▶ continue as directed by the voice/visual prompts.

Figure 2.13 The use of an AED

Link

See page 87 for more information on the safe airway position.

Quick check

What you would check for, and how might you prepare, a casualty's chest prior to applying the defibrillator pads?

Procedure following defibrillation

Continue to follow the AED prompts until:

▷ qualified help arrives and takes over, OR

▷ the victim starts to show signs of regaining consciousness, such as coughing, opening their eyes, speaking or moving purposefully AND starts to breathe normally, OR

▷ you become exhausted.

Following successful resuscitation, repeat the primary survey and continue to the secondary survey (see pages 42 and 67).

Turn the casualty on their side into the safe airway position if they start breathing effectively but remain unconscious.

Leave the pads in place and the defibrillator on as it will continue to analyse the heart rhythm. Record the sequence and number of shocks delivered or shocks not-advised.

Advanced decision and DNA-CPRs

Some casualties may have either an Advanced Decision (sometimes referred to as a 'living will') or a 'Do Not Attempt CPR' (DNA-CPR) order in place. Both are methods of expressing a particular wish for a form of treatment to take place at some time in the future while the individual is able to express a preference they would not be able to if they were to become unwell, with a condition such as cardiac arrest or collapse. Typically this is made by individuals with terminal illnesses who do not want treatment to sustain life, such as CPR. The Advanced Decision may include some treatments but not others, or may relate to particular situations.

A DNA-CPR is a form of Advanced Decision that solely relates to the individual's decision to refuse CPR in the future.

Both Advanced Decisions and DNA-CPRs are legally binding as long as the casualty had mental capacity at the time of writing, and as long as they are within date, apply to the situation and are signed by the individual and a witness.

Application of an Advanced Decision or DNA-CPR

If the casualty is found to be unconscious and not breathing or not breathing normally, CPR should be initiated unless:

▶ a formal, written DNA-CPR is in place and handed to yourself or verbally received and recorded by ambulance control from the casualty's attendant requesting the ambulance, providing that:
  - the order is seen and corroborated by the ambulance staff on arrival
  - the condition to resuscitate relates to the condition for which the Order is in force; CPR should not be withheld for coincidental conditions.

▶ the casualty is in the final stages of terminal illness where death is imminent and unavoidable and CPR would not be successful.

In a pre-hospital setting there may be doubt as to the validity of an Advanced Decision or DNA-CPR, especially if a written document cannot be produced. If you are not satisfied that the casualty has made an Advanced Decision or has a DNA-CPR in place, you should continue to resuscitate.

Assessment practice 2.4   (C, EC) 1.1, 2.1, 2.2

You are called to an 87-year-old male who has collapsed after complaining of chest pain. You are in an urban environment with your complete medic bag.

1 What would be your initial actions for managing this casualty?

2 How would your actions differ if you were assisted by a colleague?

Understanding the recognition and management of life extinct

Upon arrival at the scene, based on the mechanism of injury or after assessing the casualty, it may be evident that resuscitation of the casualty may not, despite best efforts, be successful. Resuscitation should be attempted for most casualties but where the following situations apply and the casualty is not breathing, resuscitation should not be attempted.

Signs	Explanation
Decapitation	The head is separated from the torso.
Massive cranial and cerebral destruction	Obvious and serious head injuries, particularly where the skull has obvious deformities as a result of injury or where the brain is exposed.
Hemicorporectomy or similar massive injury	Hemicorporectomy is where the torso has been separated above the pelvis. Other massive injuries to the chest and abdomen, especially where organs are external to the body, are not considered compatible with life.
Incineration	Charred remains or greater than 95% full thickness burns.
Rigor mortis	A few hours after death, limbs will begin to stiffen; this may last 1–4 days before limbs will begin to relax again. The exception to this rule is hypothermia, which will also cause limbs to stiffen but is not, in the hypothermic casualty, a sign of life extinct.
Decomposition/ putrefaction	When the casualty has been dead for an extended period of time, the body will begin to decay.

Actions to be taken following the establishment of life extinct

The management of the body and the scene will vary depending upon whether the death occurs in public or private and whether the death is suspicious or not.

Expected death in a non-public place

▶ With an expected death in a private setting, the police would not normally be required to attend as long as end-of-life arrangements can be confirmed.

▶ Liaise with the family/carer to contact the preferred funeral director.

▶ Notify Ambulance Control that police are not required to attend.

▶ Notify the casualty's GP according to local mechanisms.

▶ The body may be left in the care of a responsible person to await the arrival of the funeral director.

▶ Complete the PRFs.

Unexpected death in a non-public place

▶ Police must be requested to attend in their capacity as the coroner's representatives – contact them via Ambulance Control.

▶ If there are no suspicious circumstances, the ambulance clinician should consider the need to remain on scene once Confirmation of Death procedure has been completed.

▶ The body may be left in the care of a responsible person, but avoid moving it.

▶ Consider the needs of the bereaved; if the relatives are well supported, it may be appropriate to complete all documentation and withdraw from the scene.

▶ Where appropriate and if available, provide bereavement literature.

▶ When leaving the scene before arrival of the police, ensure a copy of the PRF and Confirmation of Death form is left with the body.

Communication of decision to bystanders/family

▶ If resuscitation has been stopped or not attempted, the family will need reassurance and will often expect an explanation.

▶ Bereavement manifests in many ways, so it can be difficult to predict how the family will respond or behave. If you are working in a healthcare capacity, you may have a bereavement support brochure or contacts you can provide.

▶ If relatives are not present at the time of death, it is the responsibility of the police to inform them.

Adult death in a public place

▶ Contact Ambulance Control to request attendance of the police.

▶ Do not move the body.

▶ Complete any local policy documentation and remain on scene until released by the police.

▶ Conveyance of the body by ambulance should only be carried out in exceptional circumstances. If confirmation of death is made when the casualty is already in the ambulance and the clinician decides to convey the deceased to hospital, advise Ambulance Control and request that the police rendezvous at the accepting hospital.

▶ On arrival at hospital, follow local procedures for handover of a deceased patient. The default is to hand over to the Emergency Department.

▶ Ensure a copy of the Confirmation of Death form and PRF are included in the handover process.

Suspicious circumstances

▶ Preserve the scene and prevent contamination.

▶ Arrange for Ambulance Control to contact the police, stating your location.

▶ Remain at the scene until you are released by the police.

▶ Complete any necessary documentation.

> **Quick tip**
>
> Where possible, dignity should be preserved for the benefit of the casualty as well as those who may be witness to the events, but not at the expense of delivering effective casualty care.

Assessment practice 2.5 · (C, EC) 2.6

You are called to a road traffic incident involving one vehicle and one adult pedestrian. The pedestrian is the only casualty, is showing no signs of life and has serious trauma.

1 Describe the situations in which you would not commence CPR.

2 What other factors would need to be considered to manage this situation?

Explore techniques used to manage the airway of casualties with a reduced level of consciousness

You can check, clear and open the airway with simple techniques such as postural drainage and the head tilt. In this section you will learn advanced interventions to manage a casualty's airway.

Clearing the airway

The easiest and quickest method of clearing the airway of an unconscious casualty is postural drainage. While this method is both fast and effective there is an obvious concern for aggravating existing injuries, especially spinal injuries. However, even

> **Link**
>
> See **Figure 2.4** Anatomy of the upper airway on page 48.

with a spinal injury, the priority is to maintain a clear and open airway; with a suction device it is possible to clear fluids from the casualty's mouth without needing to move the casualty or if the casualty is stabilised on a spinal board or stretcher.

Principles of suction

Suction is a relatively simple technique but exercise caution when using it. Aggressive or inappropriate suctioning can cause damage or further complications.

▶ **You must be able to visualise the airway**
This requires good lighting; this is normally the case indoors with normal room lighting or outdoors in daylight, but in low-light conditions a torch is required. A head torch is an ideal solution. If you cannot see inside the casualty's mouth, you risk causing damage by sucking the soft tissue (especially the uvula) or stimulating the gag reflex. In addition, aggressively massaging the vagus nerve at the back of the throat can lower the pulse (**bradycardia**), which can cause problems in a casualty with an already lowered pulse rate.

▶ **Aim for the corner of the mouth**
With good visibility, aim the tip of the suction catheter for the corners of the cheek behind the molars, where fluid will collect. Suctioning here avoids the soft tissue at the back of the throat, the gag reflex and the vagus nerve.

▶ **Suction on the way OUT**
Only start suctioning once the tip of the catheter is in place to avoid accidentally suctioning any soft tissue as you enter. Position the catheter first and then suction as you withdraw.

▶ **Suction for only 10 seconds at a time**
Once the airway has been cleared there is no further benefit from continuing suction. Once fluid has been removed you are now suctioning fresh air (21 per cent oxygen) from the mouth, potentially de-oxygenating the casualty. If the airway requires a lot of sustained suction, suction in phases allowing a gap between each 10-second phase.

Opening the airway

On page 50 you learned how to open the airway of an adult or child using the head tilt and neutral alignment for an infant. These are simple and effective techniques, but with trauma casualties for whom the mechanism of injury suggests spinal injury, the jaw thrust technique is used to open the casualty's airway as this method causes less movement of the spine.

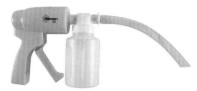
A typical manual suction unit

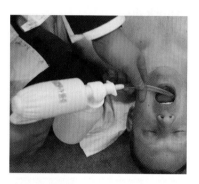

Quick check

What are the pros and cons of suctioning versus manual drainage?

The jaw thrust   `7 Steps`

1 Kneeling at the casualty's head, place your thumbs on the casualty's cheek bones.

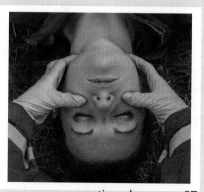

continued on page 87

The jaw thrust (*continued*)

2 With your index fingers, open the casualty's mouth to ensure it is clear.

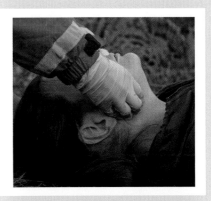

3 If there is fluid in the airway, use suction to clear the airway if suction is available. If suction is not available, employ postural drainage to clear the airway.

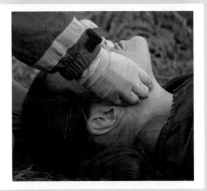

4 If there is no airway obstruction, place your third, fourth and little fingers behind the casualty's jaw, below the earlobe.

5 Pull the casualty's lower jaw up so that their lower jaw is above their upper jaw.

6 Using your index fingers again, close the casualty's mouth.

7 Maintain a grip on the casualty's jaw – letting go will immediately close the casualty's airway.

There are a number of problems associated with the jaw thrust.

▸ The jaw thrust is a two-handed technique – while applying the jaw thrust the responder's hands are tied.

▸ Applying the jaw thrust is tiring and difficult to maintain for long.

▸ As soon as the hands are released, the airway will close.

▸ With a jaw thrust applied, oral airways (see next) cannot be inserted.

Maintaining the airway

With the casualty's airway cleared and opened, it must be maintained. If no equipment is available, the casualty is moved into the safe airway position.

The safe airway position

1 If you have not already emptied the casualty's pockets as part of the secondary survey, do so now.

2 Kneeling next to the casualty, bring the arm closest to you out to their side. This prevents the casualty from being rolled over their arm.

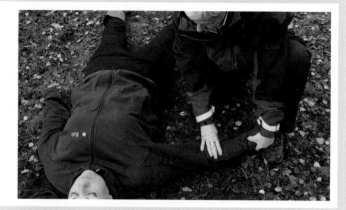

3 Reach across the casualty and lift their far leg up. This will act as a lever. As the casualty is unconscious, their leg will drop as soon as you let go, so keep control of this leg. Sometimes the foot will slide out, especially if they are lying on a shiny surface such as tiles or a wet surface. In this instance taking the foot of their elevated leg under the knee of the leg closest to you can help resolve this.

4 With the other hand, reach across to the casualty's far hand. Link your thumb with their thumb.

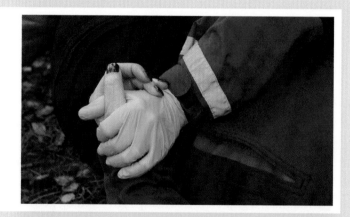

5 Bring their arm across their chest.

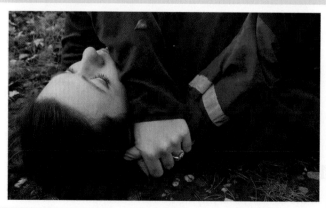

continued on page 87

The safe airway position (*continued*)

6 Maintaining control of their far hand with your thumb, open your fingers and position them (along with their far hand) under the casualty's neck to support the head and pull the casualty's elevated knee towards you.

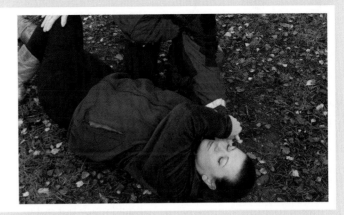

7 All of the rolling effort should be done with the knee. As soon as the casualty's far hip is off the floor the casualty should continue to roll towards you with little effort.

8 Support the casualty's head as they roll towards you.

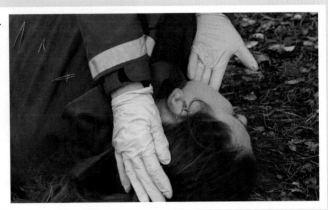

9 Continue to roll the casualty until the elbow of the arm you are controlling touches the floor. If you position the casualty before this stage, there is a risk they could roll onto their back if left unattended.

There is a potential for pressure sores to develop if the casualty is left in this position on a hard surface, in which case roll the casualty back onto their back and reposition them in the safe airway position on their other side every 30 minutes until help arrives.

Airway adjuncts

The safe airway position is a basic and essential skill for all first aiders but, again, the movement of the casualty is a cause for concern for casualties with trauma, especially spinal injury. Airway adjuncts are simple devices that can keep the unconscious casualty's airway open while they are on their back.

Warning: Both airway adjuncts described next maintain an open airway but neither will prevent fluids from building up in the airway. Just because an airway adjunct has been inserted does not mean that the airway will remain clear. Maintain regular assessment of the airway and breathing and if you suspect the airway has become or is becoming **occluded**, take immediate action to clear the airway if required.

Key term

Occluded – blocked or obstructed.

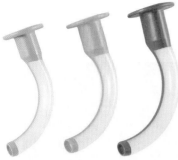

A selection of different sized OPAs

Oropharyngeal airway

The oropharyngeal airway (also known as an OPA or oral airway) is a simple plastic tube that is placed in the casualty's mouth and sits behind the tongue, preventing the relaxed tongue of an unconscious casualty from dropping back and blocking their airway.

As with suction, these simple items need to be applied and fitted appropriately and safely to avoid damage and further complications.

Assessing the casualty

A casualty who you intend to insert an OPA in must be unresponsive or not breathing. Any casualty with a response (to either voice or pain) has a gag reflex. Attempting to insert an OPA into a casualty may cause them to gag, vomit, reject or resist the OPA.

Sizing the OPA

Place the flange of the OPA on the centre of the casualty's mouth. The end of the OPA should reach but not extend beyond the angle of the casualty's jaw.

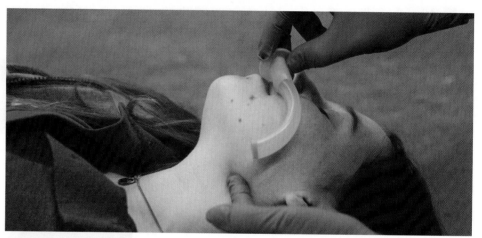

Place the OPA against the casualty's cheek from the centre of their mouth to the angle of the jaw

Inserting the OPA

Rotate the OPA upside down before inserting into the casualty's mouth. Attempting to insert the OPA in its normal orientation is likely to push the tongue back, blocking the casualty's airway. Rotate the OPA through 90 degrees as you progress the OPA inwards. Continue to rotate through 90 degrees as you continue to fully insert the OPA.

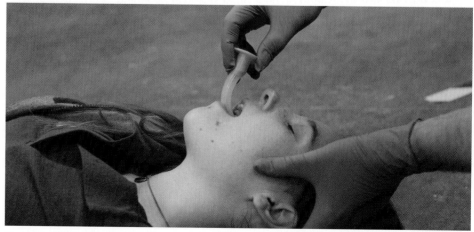

Place the OPA upside down initially

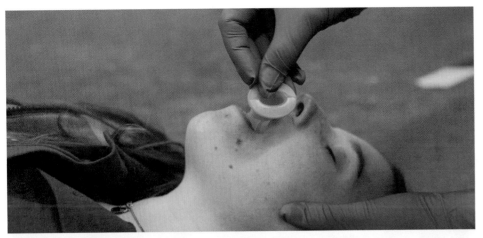

Rotate the OPA 90 degrees as it is introduced into the mouth

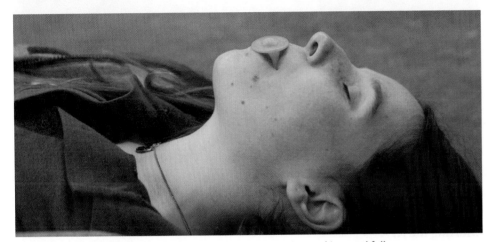

Continue to rotate the OPA until it is in the correct orientation and inserted fully

Children and infants

Children and infants have a delicate soft palate; as such, the OPA should be introduced in the normal orientation using a tongue depressor to depress the tongue during insertion.

Check the casualty to ensure they are still breathing. If breathing is absent, remove the OPA, reassess breathing and attempt again.

Removing the OPA

The OPA comes out in the same orientation; there is no need to rotate the OPA as you withdraw it.

Nasopharyngeal airway

The nasopharyngeal airway (NPA or nasal airway) is a soft flexible tube that is inserted into an unconscious casualty's nostril – into the nasopharynx and down behind the oropharynx, where it sits behind the tongue, preventing it from falling back and blocking their airway of an unconscious casualty. One of the benefits of the NPA over the OPA is that the casualty does not need to be unresponsive; an NPA may be inserted into a casualty who is unconscious but responding to voice or pain. As the NPA is less likely to stimulate the gag reflex it is better tolerated by a wider range of casualties. Furthermore, the unresponsive casualty who has had an OPA inserted may not remain unresponsive; if they become responsive they are likely to gag or reject the airway. An unresponsive casualty with an NPA fitted is less likely to do this.

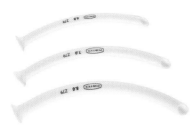

A selection of different sized NPAs

Assessing the casualty

An NPA can be inserted in to any unconscious casualty who may still be responsive but not fully alert.

Sizing the NPA

Place the flange against the nostril of the casualty. The tip should reach, but not extend beyond, the angle of the jaw.

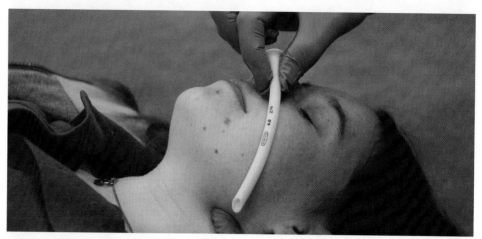

Place the NPA against the casualty's cheek from the nostril to the angle of the jaw

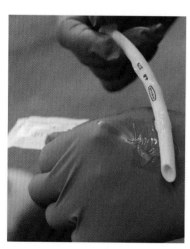

Lubricate the NPA

Preparing the NPA

Unlike the OPA, the NPA should be lubricated with a water-based lubricant before insertion. This is best achieved by applying a small amount of lubricant to the back of a gloved hand and wiping the NPA through it. This prevents getting lubricant on your fingers and contaminating the rest of your equipment.

Inserting the NPA

▶ NPAs are designed to be placed in the right nostril as standard.

▶ Kneel on the right of the casualty and with your left hand on the casualty's forehead, holding the airway open, use your left thumb to pull back the tip of the nose, this opens the nostrils making insertion easier.

▶ Align the bevel of the NPA against the septum.

▶ Hold the NPA vertically and slowly introduce the NPA. If resistance is felt, do not force the NPA; remove it and attempt to insert in the left nostril.

▶ Insert the NPA until the flange is flush with the casualty's nostril.

▶ Assess the casualty's breathing.

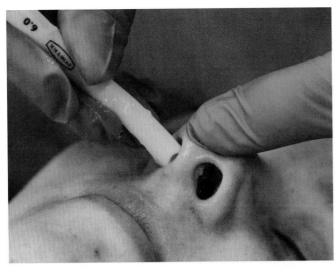

1 Correct orientation of the NPA – notice the bevel is aligned to the casualty's septum

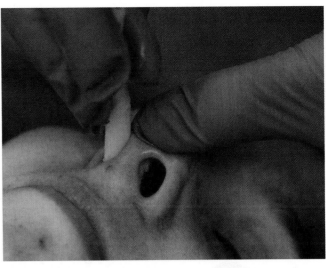

2 The NPA is inserted vertically – opening the nostrils can aid insertion

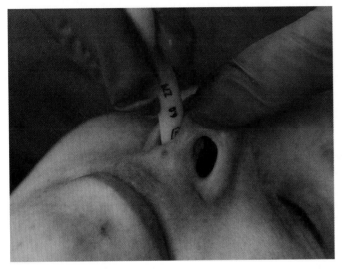

3 Push down gently

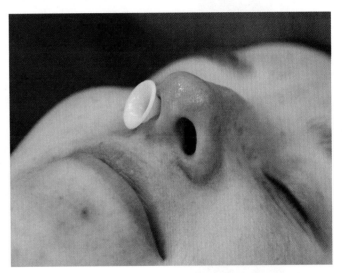

4 The NPA is inserted until the flange is flush with the nostril

Removing the NPA

The NPA is simply withdrawn from the casualty's nostril.

Assessment practice 2.6

(C, EC) 3.9

The casualty you are called to is an unconscious female who is responding to pain. She has collapsed suddenly with no sign of injury. She is breathing but her breathing is weak.

1 What options do you have to maintain her airway?

2 Describe the pros and cons for each.

Explore the provision of supplemental oxygen

Key term

Hypoxia – a lack of oxygen reaching the tissues.

Oxygen is fundamental to sustaining life or, more accurately, the right amount of oxygen is fundamental in sustaining life. It is typical for casualties to suffer from **hypoxia**, due to problems with their airway, breathing or circulation caused by either injury or illness. Too much oxygen, however, can also cause problems. You need to know how much oxygen to give a casualty and how to give it to them. With oxygen, more is not always better.

Before you deliver supplemental oxygen, you need to be familiar with the equipment available to you and how to use it safely and appropriately.

Oxygen cylinders

Oxygen cylinders contain approximately 100 per cent oxygen at extremely high pressures, so there are inherent risks whenever you use supplementary oxygen. Before an oxygen cylinder is used, the following checks should be made.

▶ **Table 2.19**

Check	Reason
Contents	Is it oxygen? Some oxygen cylinders are clearly labelled, others are colour coded. In the UK most oxygen cylinders are black with white shoulders, but some are all white. In the USA oxygen cylinders are green. Before you give the casualty oxygen, make sure you are giving them oxygen!
Damage	A cylinder is an inherently strong shape as pressure is distributed evenly around the curve. Any dents in the cylinder are weak spots. Aside from superficial damage such as scuffs and scratches, are there any dents? Is the mechanism clean and functioning? Is the pressure gauge cracked?
Pressure	Is there enough oxygen in the cylinder? A half-used cylinder can be used but if the needle is in the red, start a new cylinder.
Date	100% oxygen does not go off but the cylinder will be marked with an expiry date – this is for the integrity of the cylinder. Cylinders left unused may corrode or seize up. Rubber o-ring seals may perish if exposed to extremes of temperature, for example.

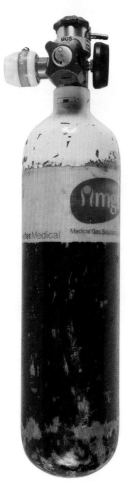

An oxygen cylinder

The oxygen cylinder may have a separate regulator that must be fitted to the top of it or the regulator may be integral to the cylinder. There are a number of features you must be familiar with:

▶ **On–off switch**
This is a high pressure valve that allows oxygen from the cylinder into the regulator.

▶ **Regulator**
This allows the oxygen out of the cylinder at various flow rates. The dial will have a number of increments from 0 litres per minute (l/min) to 15 l/min.

▶ **Outlet**
This is a barbed 'fir tree' nozzle from where the oxygen leaves the cylinder. To this, you will attach the oxygen tubing of the delivery device you want to use.

Delivery devices

One way you can vary the amount of oxygen you give to a casualty is by selecting the flow rate on the cylinder; the other is by choosing the appropriate delivery device. There are various delivery devices available and each serves a particular purpose.

Bag-valve-mask

The BVM is used to ventilate a casualty who is not breathing as it forces air into the casualty's lungs. It can be used on its own to provide 21 per cent oxygen from the atmosphere or it can be connected to an oxygen cylinder to deliver up to 100 per cent oxygen. When connected to an oxygen cylinder, the oxygen inflates the reservoir bag, ensuring a constant supply of oxygen.

The BVM is usually delivered with 12–15 l/min.

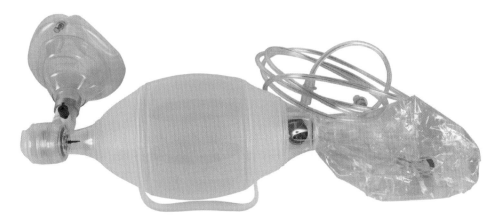

Non-rebreather mask

For a casualty who is breathing, a non-rebreather mask can supply high concentrations of oxygen to critically ill casualties. The non-rebreather mask is so called because it draws on a reservoir or oxygen (supplied from the oxygen cylinder) that passes through a one-way valve. This valve allows oxygen into the casualty as they inhale but closes as they exhale into the mask, preventing expired carbon dioxide entering the reservoir and diluting the oxygen concentration. Exhaled air leaves the mask through one-way valves on the side, which close on inhalation preventing atmospheric air (at only 21 per cent) from entering the mask and diluting the oxygen concentration.

Quick tip

Place your finger over the inlet valve of the non-rebreather mask to speed up the inflation of the reservoir bag before giving it to the casualty.

Warning: Before the non-rebreather mask is given to the casualty, ensure the reservoir bag is filled with oxygen.

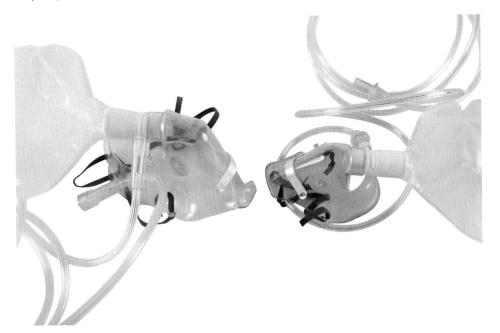

The non-rebreather mask can deliver around 85–95 per cent oxygen. The slight loss of concentration is due to leaks between the mask and the face (which is almost impossible to completely eradicate) and the small amount of exhaled carbon dioxide that does not vent out of the mask before the next inhalation.

A non-rebreather mask is usually delivered with 10–15 l/min. Below this there is not enough pressure to remove exhaled carbon dioxide from the mask.

Simple face mask

A simple face mask is for casualties who require a moderate amount of oxygen. It is similar to the non-rebreather mask but it does not have the reservoir bag, so the casualty is breathing in oxygen as it comes from the cylinder. Exhaled air escapes through holes in the side of the mask. As there is no reservoir or valves, this mask will provide around 35–65 per cent oxygen at 8–12 l/min.

Pocket mask

The pocket mask is used to assist mouth-to-mouth ventilation during CPR. Used on its own it allows the first responder to exhale 16 per cent oxygen into the casualty. The pocket mask has an inlet port to connect to the oxygen cylinder. At 15 l/min the supplemental oxygen allows the responder to exhale a combination of approximately 50 per cent oxygen into the casualty.

Venturi mask

The venturi mask is a specialised piece of equipment for critically ill casualties who require a very specific amount of oxygen, such as those with chronic obstructive pulmonary disorder (COPD). It is difficult to ascertain accurately what concentrations of oxygen casualties receive with the non-rebreather and normal mask. The venturi mask features an adjustable venturi barrel with different sized holes or replaceable ports of different sizes, allowing a specified amount of air to mix with the oxygen. The venturi mask is able to administer 24–60 per cent oxygen at 4–10 l/min.

Nasal cannula

The nasal cannula comprises a tube with prongs that sit inside the nostrils of casualties who only require low levels of supplementary oxygen. The nasal mask can deliver 24–44 per cent oxygen at 2–6 l/min.

Tracheostomy mask

A tracheostomy mask is a contoured mask designed to make a seal over a casualty's stoma for the provision of supplementary oxygen. The mask features a standard 22 mm fitting for attachment to a bag-valve mask or venturi adapter.

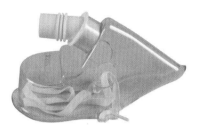

A simple face mask

Link

For more information on COPD, see page 98 and Unit 4, page 163.

Link

See Modifications for neck breathers on page 79.

Quick tip

If a tracheostomy mask is not available, a paediatric-sized face mask can be used to make a seal over the stoma.

Assessing the need for supplementary oxygen

The casualty's vital signs will give you an immediate indication of their need for supplementary oxygen.

▶ **Table 2.20**

Vital sign	Indication
Level of response	A reduction of oxygen to the brain will reduce the casualty's level of response as the brain is no longer able to function normally.
Breathing	A casualty with difficulty breathing will not be getting as much oxygen as they normally would.
Colour	Oxygen bound to red blood cells causes the blood cells to look bright red; a lack of oxygen causes the blood to look dark red, but through the skin this will look blue, like veins. Blueness to the lips (cyanosis) is a clear sign of a lack of oxygen.

All of the earlier signs indicate a need for oxygen but they do not tell us how much to give. How much oxygen you administer depends on either the cause, or the casualty's oxygen saturation levels.

▶ Any casualty in cardiac arrest will receive 15 l/min via the bag-valve mask.

▶ Any breathing casualty injured as a result of trauma will receive 15 l/min via a non-rebreather mask.

▶ Any other breathing casualty will receive oxygen based on their oxygen saturation levels.

▶ All casualties with COPD require a specific amount of oxygen.

Oxygen saturation

Oxygen saturation is measured as a percentage of red blood cells with oxygen bound to them. Each red blood cell can carry four oxygen molecules, so, in theory, if all of your red blood cells had four oxygen molecules bound to them, your oxygen saturation (or SpO_2) would be 100 per cent.

To measure a casualty's oxygen saturation, a pulse oximeter is used. The term SpO_2 comes from the measurement of peripheral oxygen saturation as it is typically measured in a pre-hospital setting at the fingertip. In hospital they may measure the oxygen saturation from samples of blood taken from the arteries – SpO_2. This is far more accurate but not practical in a pre-hospital setting.

Using a pulse oximeter

The pulse oximeter will either be a single unit that clips onto the finger like a clothes peg, or the sensor will clip to the finger and the digital readout will be separate, attached by a lead.

When the unit is turned on, a red light will be seen inside the sensor; this must be placed directly over the casualty's fingernail. The unit will display both the casualty's pulse, in beats per minute, and their SpO_2 as a percentage. This simple device is the only way of measuring a casualty's oxygen saturation but its accuracy can depend on a number of factors:

▶ Nail varnish or false nails will reduce the reading.

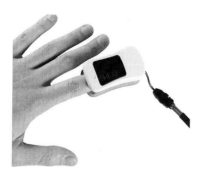

A typical pulse oximeter

Link

See Unit 4, page 163, for more information on COPD.

Key term

Titrating – continuously measuring and adjusting the balance of drug dosage.

- Cold casualties or hypovolaemic casualties with poor peripheral circulation may not detect a reading.
- Shivering or movement might affect the reading.
- Bright, overhead light may give a false, higher reading.
- Carbon monoxide poisoning will also give a high reading because the pulse oximeter cannot differentiate red blood cells bound to oxygen from red blood cells bound to CO.
- Irregular heart rhythms may cause failure to detect a reading.

While full oxygen saturation levels would be 100 per cent, that is not actually normal. Most people have an SpO$_2$ somewhere between 94 per cent and 99 per cent. Below 94 per cent SpO$_2$ the casualty is said to be hypoxic. Below 90 per cent the casualty is considered to be severely hypoxic.

Chronic obstructive pulmonary disorders

Casualties with COPD (including asthma, bronchitis and emphysema) are used to living with lower oxygen saturation; as such they require less supplemental oxygen than you would normally give to other casualties. Where a healthy person would typically have oxygen saturation of over 94 per cent breathing normal air, a COPD patient would normally have saturation of 88–92 per cent; you should aim to oxygenate to that level. Moderating oxygen flow to a target saturation level – **titrating** – has been seen to reduce mortality by 58 per cent compared to using high-flow oxygen for casualties with COPD. These casualties require a very specific amount of oxygen.

Summary

The amount of oxygen administered depends on the cause or the oxygen saturation levels. How much you give, and how you give it, will be determined by the flow rate and the delivery device.

▶ **Table 2.21**

Casualty	Flow rate	Delivery device	Target saturation
Not breathing	15 l/min	Bag-valve mask	SpO$_2$ 94%+
Any serious trauma or SpO$_2$ <85%	10–15 l/min	Non-rebreather mask	
Any other casualty SpO$_2$ 85–93%	2–6 l/min	Nasal cannula	
COPD	4 l/min	28% Venturi mask	SpO$_2$ 88–92%
	1–2 l/min	Nasal cannula	

Administering supplemental oxygen

Quick tip

When opening or closing the oxygen cylinder, turn the dial back a quarter of a turn to prevent it from seizing up in that position.

- Check the oxygen cylinder for:
  - contents
  - damage
  - pressure
  - date.
- Ensure the regulator is set to zero before opening the cylinder.
- Turn the on-off valve all the way to open.
- Open the regulator all of the way to 15 l/min (or maximum amount available) to blow out any dust or debris that may be in the outlet nozzle. Return the regulator to zero.
- Select the appropriate mask for the condition of the casualty.
- Connect the oxygen tube to the outlet nozzle of the oxygen cylinder.

▸ Open the regulator to the desired flow rate.
  - If using the non-rebreather mask or bag-valve mask, ensure the reservoir bag is inflated before administering the oxygen to the casualty.

▸ If the casualty is conscious:
  - explain to them what you are doing; do not force a mask onto a casualty's face without explaining what you are doing and why
  - explain that oxygen from the cylinder is very dry and they may notice their nose or throat feeling dry as a result.

▸ After use, return the regulator to zero and close the on–off switch.

Safety considerations

Oxygen is not flammable but it supports combustion. The Fire Triangle reminds us that fire requires heat, fuel and oxygen; therefore if there is any fuel in the presence of heat while concentrated oxygen is being used, a fire is a real risk.

> **Quick tip**
>
> If administering oxygen to an infant, tape the infant's eyes closed to prevent the oxygen escaping from the mask from damaging the mucous membrane around the infant's eyes.

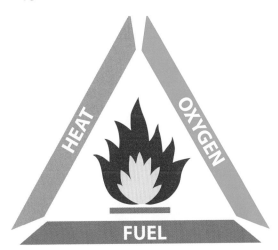

Figure 2.14 The Fire Triangle shows the elements required to create fire

Sources of heat or ignition include fire, embers, lit cigarettes or other ignition sources such as electrical equipment that may spark. A pacemaker fitted to the casualty is not a source of ignition. There is a very low risk of an AED creating a spark as the electrodes are adhesive and ensuring good pad contact means there is no gap for the electricity to 'arc' across. When a casualty is being defibrillated, simply remove the delivery device to 1 m away.

Sources of fuel include any combustible materials, such as oils and greases. Hydrocarbon-based oils and grease do not need an ignition source if the oxygen supplied is highly concentrated and under high pressure. For this reason, hands, gloves and the regulator must be free from oil and grease before use.

Assessment practice 2.7 (C, EC) 5.1

You are called to a casualty who is known to have emphysema. On arrival they have obvious difficulty breathing.

1. Does this casualty require supplementary oxygen?
2. How could you confirm this?
3. Describe the equipment you would use and which flow rates would be best to treat this casualty.

Further reading and resources

Pilberry, R. and Lethbridge, K., Ambulance Care Essentials, Brigg, United Kingdom, Class Publishing, 2015.

Association of Ambulance Chief Executives, UK Ambulance Services Clinical Practice Guidelines, Bridgwater, United Kingdom, Class Publishing, 2016.

Websites

fphc.rcsed.ac.uk
Consensus Statements from the Royal College of Surgeons of Edinburgh, Faculty of Pre-hospital Care

www.hse.gov.uk
Health and Safety Executive guidance on manual handling

www.resus.org.uk
Latest guidelines for UK resuscitation protocols and manual handling guidance

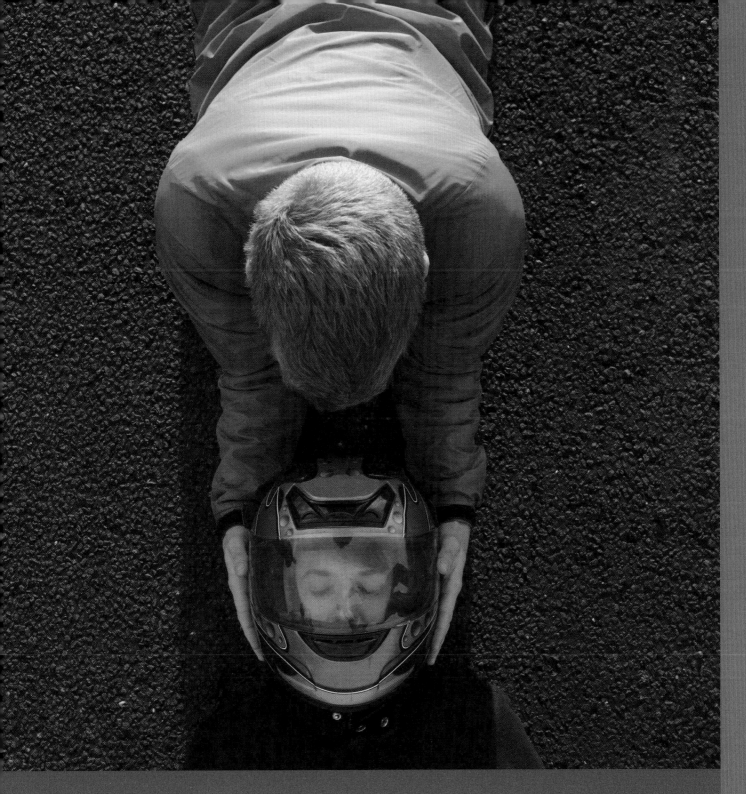

Recognising and
Managing Trauma for
the First Responder

3

Getting to know your unit

Casualties that the first responder is likely to encounter include those who have suffered traumatic injuries. From casualties who have fallen from height to those suffering from burns, the first responder needs to be able to effectively assess, recognise and manage the casualty suffering a traumatic injury or illness before handing over to definitive pre-hospital care providers.

In this unit you will learn how to recognise and manage the trauma casualty who may have suffered thermal injuries, exposure, drowning, musculoskeletal injuries, head injuries, spinal injuries or chest injuries. You will learn how to recognise and manage a casualty suffering with hypovolaemic shock, the different types of bleeding and how to manage these casualties. You will also develop an understanding of how to apply correct manual handling to prevent injury to yourself and the casualty, as well as how to package the casualty appropriately ready for transfer.

During the unit, you will not only develop your knowledge and understanding in a theoretical context but also, in simulated environments, you will practically explore the principles and techniques used by the first responder to recognise and manage casualties with trauma-related injuries or conditions. This will begin to prepare you for the final synoptic unit in which your ability to manage incidents involving casualties requiring trauma care competently will be assessed.

How you will be assessed

This unit will comprise a series of internally assessed tasks set by your centre. How they perform this assessment will vary from centre to centre. Throughout the unit there are assessment practice activities to help you work towards your assessment. Completing these will not mean you have achieved a Pass or Fail, but that you have carried out useful research and preparation.

In order to achieve a Pass, you need to meet all the Assessment criteria. The assessment set by your centre will comprise a number of tasks designed to meet the criteria in the following tables. This is likely to consist of a written assignment but may also include activities such as:

▶ producing a guide book about the recognition and management of trauma casualties

▶ producing a video guide to demonstrate applying/removing collars or helmets

▶ creating a presentation, video or leaflet on manual handling and casualty extrication.

How the unit is covered: This unit's Learning outcomes and Assessment criteria differ between the Certificate and the Extended Certificate specifications in their order and criteria wording. As elsewhere in the book, the content of the unit aligns with the order of the Extended Certificate. If you are studying the Certificate specification, look at Table 3.1 for details of the outcomes and criteria you are expected to meet.

Unit 3 Learning outcomes and Assessment criteria (Certificate)

▶ **Table 3.1**

Learning outcome 1: Understand the recognition and management of casualties with burns

Assessment criteria	
1.1	Describe the signs and symptoms of different severities of burns
1.2	Identify the different hazardous material warning signs
1.3	Explain the management of a casualty with a dry burn or scald
1.4	Explain how and why management plans vary for casualties with special types of burn

Learning outcome 2: Understand the recognition and management of casualties with hypothermia and hyperthermia

Assessment criteria	
2.1	Describe the signs and symptoms of hypothermia and hyperthermia
2.2	Describe the stages of hypothermia and hyperthermia
2.3	Explain the management of casualties suffering from hypothermia and hyperthermia

Learning outcome 3: Understand the recognition and management of casualties with musculoskeletal injuries

Assessment criteria	
3.1	Describe the different types of fracture
3.2	Describe the signs and symptoms of a possible fracture or dislocation
3.3	Explain the management of a casualty with a possible open fracture
3.4	Explain the management of a casualty with a possible closed fracture
3.5	Explain the management of a casualty with a possible dislocation
3.6	Describe the signs and symptoms of a sprain or strain
3.7	Explain the management of casualties with a possible strain or strain
3.8	Explain the management of a casualty with a possible pelvic fracture
3.9	Explain the management of a casualty with a possible chest injury

Learning outcome 4: Understand the recognition and management of casualties with a head injury

Assessment criteria	
4.1	Explain four mechanisms of injury that have potential to cause a head injury
4.2	Describe the signs and symptoms of a minor head injury
4.3	Explain the management of a casualty with a minor head injury
4.4	Describe the signs and symptoms of a casualty with a potentially serious head injury
4.5	Explain the management of a casualty with a potentially serious head injury

Learning outcome 5: Understand the recognition and management of a casualty with a spinal injury

Assessment criteria	
5.1	Explain four mechanisms of injury that may cause spinal trauma
5.2	Describe the signs and symptoms of a casualty with a suspected spinal injury
5.3	Explain the management of a casualty with a suspected spinal injury

Learning outcome 6: Understand the recognition and management of casualties with wounds and bleeding

Assessment criteria	
6.1	Describe three different types of wound
6.2	Describe signs and symptoms of internal blood loss
6.3	Explain the management of casualties with a non-compressible haemorrhage
6.4	Explain the management of a casualty with a compressible haemorrhage
6.5	Explain the management of an amputated limb
6.6	Explain the special considerations for the management of a casualty suffering from a facial injury
6.7	Explain the management of a casualty with a nose bleed

Learning outcome 7: Understand the recognition and management of a casualty suffering from hypovolaemic shock

Assessment criteria	
7.1	Describe the stages of hypovolaemic shock
7.2	Explain the management of casualties suffering from hypovolaemic shock

Learning outcome 8: Understand the principles of manual handling

Assessment criteria	
8.1	Explain how two types of manual handling injury can occur
8.2	Explain the TILE(O) system for dynamic manual handling risk assessment
8.3	Describe the principles of correct manual handling techniques for lifting
8.4	Describe the principles of correct manual handling techniques for pushing and pulling
8.5	Explain the three methods of transferring a casualty in cardiorespiratory arrest from chair to floor
8.6	Explain the importance of appropriate manual handling techniques to the first responder

Unit 3 Learning outcomes and Assessment criteria (Extended Certificate)

▶ **Table 3.2**

Learning outcome 1: Understand the recognition and management of casualties with burns

Assessment criteria	
1.1	Describe the signs and symptoms of different severities of burns
1.2	Identify the different hazardous material warning signs
1.3	Explain the management of a casualty with a dry burn or scald
1.4	Explain how and why management plans vary for casualties with special types of burn

Learning outcome 2: Understand the recognition and management of casualties with hypothermia and hyperthermia and their related injuries

Assessment criteria

2.1	Describe the signs and symptoms of hypothermia and hyperthermia
2.2	Describe the stages of hypothermia and hyperthermia
2.3	Explain the management of casualties suffering from hypothermia and hyperthermia
2.4	Describe the signs and symptoms of casualties suffering from cold injuries
2.5	Explain the management of casualties suffering from cold injuries
2.6	Explain the special considerations when handling casualties exposed to extremes of temperature in austere environments

Learning outcome 3: Understand the recognition and management of the conscious near drowned casualty

Assessment criteria

| 3.1 | Describe the signs and symptoms of a conscious casualty following a near drowning |
| 3.2 | Explain the management of a conscious near drowning casualty |

Learning outcome 4: Understand the recognition and management of casualties with musculoskeletal injuries

Assessment criteria

4.1	Describe the different types of fracture
4.2	Describe the signs and symptoms of a possible fracture or dislocation
4.3	Explain the management of a casualty with a possible open fracture
4.4	Explain the management of a casualty with a possible closed fracture
4.5	Explain the management of a casualty with a possible dislocation
4.6	Describe the signs and symptoms of a sprain or strain
4.7	Explain the management of a casualty with a possible pelvic fracture
4.8	Explain the management of casualties with a possible sprain or strain
4.9	Describe the components of a basic joint examination
4.10	Describe the features of a limb which has a circulation compromise
4.11	Explain the management of a limb with a circulation compromise

Learning outcome 5: Understand the recognition and management of casualties with a head injury

Assessment criteria

5.1	Explain four mechanisms of injury that have potential to cause a head injury
5.2	Describe the signs and symptoms of a minor head injury
5.3	Explain the management of a casualty with a minor head injury
5.4	Describe the signs and symptoms of a casualty with a potentially serious head injury
5.5	Explain the management of a casualty with a potentially serious head injury

Learning outcome 6: Explore the recognition and management of a casualty with a spinal injury

Assessment criteria

| 6.1 | Explain four mechanisms of injury that may cause spinal trauma |
| 6.2 | Describe the signs and symptoms of a casualty with a suspected spinal injury |

6.3	Explain the management of a casualty with a suspected spinal injury
6.4	Explain the application of a rigid cervical collar for a casualty with a suspected spinal injury
6.5	Demonstrate the application of a rigid cervical collar for a casualty with a suspected spinal injury
6.6	Explain the removal of helmets from a casualty with a suspected spinal injury
6.7	Demonstrate the removal of a helmet from a casualty with a suspected spinal injury

Learning outcome 7: Understand the recognition and management of casualties with wounds and bleeding

Assessment criteria

7.1	Describe three different types of wound
7.2	Describe the signs and symptoms of internal blood loss
7.3	Explain the management of casualties with a non-compressible haemorrhage
7.4	Explain the management of a casualty with a compressible haemorrhage
7.5	Explain the management of an amputated limb
7.6	Explain the special considerations for the management of a casualty suffering from a facial injury
7.7	Explain the special considerations for the management of a casualty suffering from a crush injury
7.8	Explain the management of a casualty with a nose bleed

Learning outcome 8: Understand the recognition and management of a casualty suffering from hypovolaemic shock

Assessment criteria

| **8.1** | Describe the stages of hypovolaemic shock |
| **8.2** | Explain the management of casualties suffering from hypovolaemic shock |

Learning outcome 9: Understand the recognition and management of casualties with chest injuries

Assessment criteria

9.1	Describe the signs and symptoms of four different chest injuries
9.2	Explain the method of conducting a chest examination for a casualty suffering with a traumatic chest injury
9.3	Explain the management of a casualty suffering from a chest wound
9.4	Compare the management of casualties suffering from other chest injuries

Learning outcome 10: Understand the principles of manual handling and casualty extraction

Assessment criteria

10.1	Explain how two types of manual handling injury can occur
10.2	Explain the TILE(O) system for dynamic manual handling risk assessment
10.3	Describe the principles of correct manual handling techniques for lifting
10.4	Describe the principles of correct manual handling techniques for pushing and pulling
10.5	Explain the three methods of transferring a casualty in cardiorespiratory arrest from chair to floor
10.6	Analyse the use of three different types of stretcher for appropriately moving casualties
10.7	Explain the importance of appropriate manual handling techniques to the first responder

As a first responder, you will encounter various types of traumatic injury for which you need to be prepared. Think about the contents of your closest first-aid kit. In which situations or environments would you use these items? Do you have sufficient and appropriate equipment to undertake any situation?

Understand the recognition and management of casualties suffering from burns

Burns and scalds damage the skin with heat. Burns are caused by a dry heat, e.g. the cooker, and scalds are caused by wet heat, e.g. boiling water or steam.

Burns can also be caused by more than just direct contact with something hot. Contact with electricity, some chemicals, friction and spending too much time in strong sunlight can all cause burns.

The signs, symptoms and management are the same whether you are treating a burn or a scald, so the term 'burn' is used to mean both.

Severity of burns

To judge the severity of the burn you must consider its depth, location and size.

Depth of burn

Burns can be split into three categories of depth: superficial, partial or full thickness. The deeper the burn penetrates the layers of skin, the more severe the burn.

▶ Superficial burns: these are the least serious of the categories. They produce some reddening (erythema) of the skin and can be very painful.

▶ Partial-thickness burns: these burns penetrate the epidermis layer of skin and begin to affect the dermis layer. This causes swelling and blisters to form on the skin. These too can be extremely painful.

▶ Full-thickness burns: these are the most serious category of burn and can be life threatening. The burn reaches deep into the skin to the subcutaneous layer and destroys nerve endings and blood vessels, meaning that full-thickness burns are not as painful as areas with superficial or partial-thickness burns.

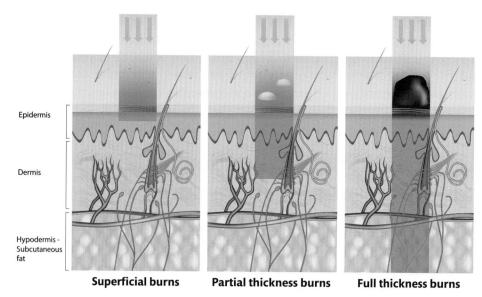

Epidermis

Dermis

Hypodermis - Subcutaneous fat

Superficial burns **Partial thickness burns** **Full thickness burns**

Figure 3.1 The layers of skin are affected in different ways depending on the severity of the burn

It is important to consider the mechanism of injury here and to consider other injuries the casualty may have. For example, if the casualty was in an enclosed environment and the burn was caused by an explosion, check whether there are any burns or damage to the casualty's airway. Do they also need to be assessed and managed for smoke inhalation? Or was the injury caused by hot water? This is more likely to run off the skin and cause less damage than hot fat, which will stick to the skin and cause a deeper injury.

Location of burn

The location of the burn on the body will also affect the severity of the burn. If the burn goes around the whole circumference of a limb or digit and is full thickness, this is a limb-threatening injury. The swelling associated with a burn can cut off the circulation to the limb and surgery will be required at hospital to release the pressure.

Burns to face, neck or genitals always require assessment at hospital. Any burns that could affect the casualty's airway will also be of higher severity; look out for soot around the mouth and nose, coughing, difficulty breathing, noisy breathing or reduced levels of consciousness. Where you suspect there is a risk of a burn to an airway, summon more qualified assistance immediately.

Size of burn

To estimate the size of a burn there are a number of different methods of which you need to be aware:

Wallace Rule of Nines: this is a quick way of estimating the surface area of the burn (see **Figures 3.2** and **3.3**).

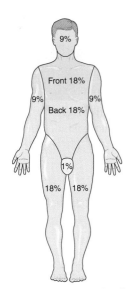

Figure 3.2 Wallace Rule of Nines: adult

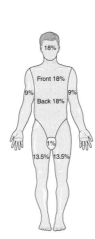

Figure 3.3 Wallace Rule of Nines: child

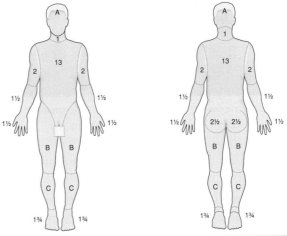

Area	Age 0	1	5	10	15	Adult
A = ½ of head	9½	8½	6½	5½	4½	3½
B = ½ of one thigh	2¾	4	4	4½	4½	4¾
C = ½ of one lower leg	2½	2¾	2¾	3	3¼	3½

Figure 3.4 Lund and Browder chart: percentage total body surface area burn

Palmar surface: the surface area of the casualty's palm, including their fingers, is approximately 1 per cent of their total body surface area. Use this to estimate the total size of the burn. This works better with smaller burns.

Lund and Browder chart: if this is used correctly, it is the most accurate as it takes into account different body shape with different ages.

Management of a burn　　`13 Steps`

1 Place the casualty in a way that they feel most comfortable.

2 Remove the casualty from the heat that caused the burn.
- Where this is a dry chemical you should wear the correct PPE and brush it off with paper towels or similar.

3 Place the burns under cool running water for 20 minutes. This ensures the affected skin is cooled and will provide some pain relief for the casualty.
- You must not use ice or iced water as this can cause further damage to the skin.
- You must be careful to keep the casualty warm while doing this to prevent hypothermia. Use a blanket or similar around the non-affected area and warm the environment the casualty is in if possible.

4 Place burns dressings on the casualty. Use these when water is not available.

5 Place sheets of cling film on to the affected area. They should never be wrapped around a limb as this can restrict swelling, causing circulatory compromise and death of the tissue in the limb.

continued on page 110

Management of a burn (*continued*)

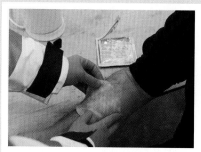

1 Place a burns dressing over the burn

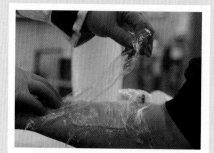

2 Place the sheets of cling film over the burn

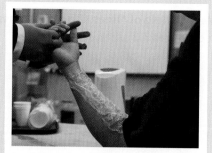

3 Ensure the cling film is not wrapped around the limb

6 Where the burn has been caused by electricity, search for entry and exit sites.

7 Ensure you document clearly the cause of the burn and what measures were taken prior to your arrival.

8 Where the burn has been caused by a chemical, note the type of chemical involved and refer to the chemical data sheet and the packaging where available.
- With chemical burns, ensure these are irrigated with lots of running water and do not dress with cling film.
- Chemicals can be absorbed into the skin and cause poisoning, so ensure you continually monitor the casualty.

9 Cut off burnt or smouldering clothing that is not stuck to the skin. Remove any close-fitting jewellery.

10 Be aware that burns can be extremely painful, so consider summoning assistance to administer pain relief where required. Also consider the cause of the burn and if you require specialist help from the fire service or the ambulance service Hazardous Area Response Team (HART).

11 Complete a full set of observations and a thorough casualty assessment.
- If you suspect a non-accidental injury with burns (especially in young children or vulnerable adults), consider if the burn area matches the history of the events given.

12 Record all of your findings and management on the Patient Report Form (PRF).

13 Hand the casualty over as required to the next echelon of pre-hospital care.

Link

See Unit 1, page 31, for more information on PRFs.

Hazardous material warning signs

Chemicals have hazard warning signs (pictograms) on their containers to let people know the dangers of the chemicals inside. These chemical hazard pictograms are required by law (Classification, Labelling and Packaging (CLP) Regulation). If there is any risk of chemical involvement in a situation to which you are called, you must check for these nine hazard pictograms. They will also be present on any chemical data sheets if these are available.

Explosives

Flammable liquids

Oxidising liquids

Compressed gases

Corrosive

Acute toxicity

Skin irritation

Aspiration hazard

Hazardous to the aquatic environment

Figure 3.5 Warning signs

Assessment practice 3.1   (C, EC) 1.1, 1.2, 1.3, 1.4

1 What are the signs and symptoms for each of the three different severities of burn?

2 List the steps you would take in the management of a superficial burn of 2 per cent to a 24-year-old's arm?

3 Identify the nine pictograms opposite.

4 How would your management of a chemical burn differ from that of a burn caused by a hot iron?

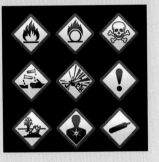

Understand the recognition and management of casualties with hypothermia, hyperthermia and their related injuries

Hypothermia

'Hypo' means low and 'thermia' refers to temperature. A casualty is hypothermic when their core body temperature drops below 35°C and this is a life-threatening condition. Hypothermia can occur in different ways and at different rates:

▶ quickly (acute hypothermia); for example when a casualty has fallen into cold water

▶ moderately quickly (subacute hypothermia); when a casualty has, for example, been out walking in cold conditions and they have become exhausted and are unable to generate enough heat to keep warm

▶ slowly (chronic hypothermia); for example, when an elderly casualty has fallen and is unable to get up, meaning they have spent a long time on the floor.

Where you suspect that a casualty is at risk of hypothermia (see **Figure 3.6**), you do not need to have gained an accurate core body temperature reading to begin management. Some people are at an increased risk, such as elderly people on particular medication who have had a fall and been rendered immobile.

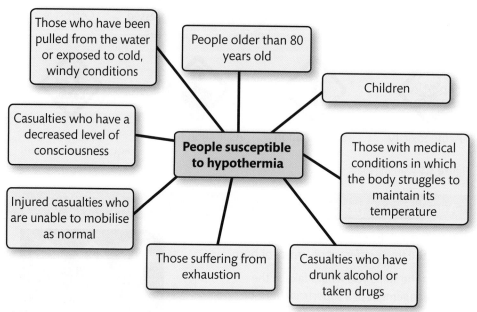

Figure 3.6 People at risk from hypothermia

Stages

Hypothermia can be sub-divided into three different stages depending on whether a casualty's core body temperature is mild, moderate or severe.

While casualties may begin to show signs of hypothermia before they reach the clinically defined core temperature of 35°C, it is important to treat them early to prevent any deterioration.

The following table shows the signs and symptoms in the stages of hypothermia.

▶ **Table 3.3**

Mild (core body temperature 35–32°C)	Moderate (core body temperature 32–28°C)	Severe (core body temperature less than 28°C)
▶ Constant shivering ▶ Fatigue ▶ Low energy ▶ Cold or pale skin ▶ Fast breathing	▶ Unable to think clearly ▶ Confusion ▶ Makes poor decisions ▶ Appears drunk ▶ Difficulty mobilising ▶ Lacks coordination ▶ Drowsiness ▶ Slurred speech ▶ Slow breathing ▶ No shivering	▶ Unconsciousness ▶ Shallow, slow breathing ▶ Weak pulses ▶ Dilated pupils ▶ Respiratory arrest ▶ Cardiac arrest

Quick tip

Those with severe symptoms should be handled very carefully due to the risk of cardiac arrest.

Management of hypothermia

`6 Steps`

1 The first, and most important, step is to prevent further heat loss from the casualty.
- Wrap the casualty up with fabric blankets then place the foil blanket over the top. Do not put foil blankets directly onto the cold skin.

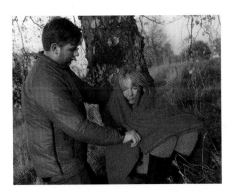 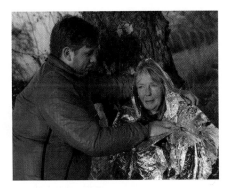

- Remove any wet clothes and wrap the casualty with blankets or dry clothing.
- Place extra layers of clothing onto the casualty if possible.

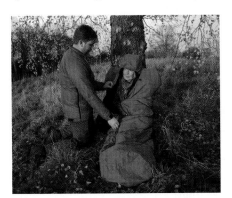 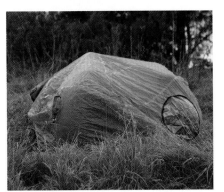

Use a wilderness survival bag and/or an emergency shelter if you have one available

- Consider moving the casualty to a warmer, more sheltered location if this is possible. Alternatively, shelter the casualty where they are, using an emergency shelter to get them out of the elements. These are particularly useful when in remote areas. If you get into the shelter with the casualty, the shelter soon warms up with your additional body heat.
- If the casualty can swallow normally and they are fully conscious, give them a warm drink.

2 Administer 100 per cent 15 lpm high-flow oxygen via a non-rebreather mask as per the guidelines.

3 Summon assistance at the earliest opportunity and consider how you are going to remove the casualty to definitive care (especially important in a remote environment).

4 Complete a full set of observations and a thorough casualty assessment.

5 Record all of your findings and management on the PRF.

6 Hand the casualty over as required to the next echelon of pre-hospital care.

Hyperthermia

Hyperthermia can be caused by external environmental factors such as the sun, or it can be caused by internal factors such as drugs or exercise.

Hyperthermia, or heat-related illness, is where the casualty is exposed to an increase in heat and can be sub-divided into three separate stages (according to the European Resuscitation Council) depending on the casualty's core body temperature.

The following table shows the three stages of hyperthermia.

Stages

▶ Table 3.4

Heat stress	Heat exhaustion (core body temperature greater than 37°C and less than 40°C)	Heat stroke (core body temperature greater than 40°C)
▶ Temperature is normal or slightly elevated ▶ Feet and ankles can become swollen ▶ **Hypotension** ▶ **Syncope** ▶ Dehydration ▶ Cramps	▶ As a result of exposure to heat over a period of hours to days ▶ Core temperature greater than 37°C and less than 40°C ▶ Headache ▶ Dizziness ▶ Nausea ▶ Vomiting ▶ **Tachycardia** ▶ Hypotension ▶ Sweating ▶ Muscle pain ▶ Cramps ▶ Reduced urination – dark in colour ▶ Thirst ▶ Tiredness and weakness	▶ Core temperature greater than 40°C ▶ Hot, dry skin ▶ Extreme fatigue ▶ Unable to coordinate ▶ Flushed ▶ Diarrhoea ▶ Decreased level of consciousness ▶ Struggling to breathe ▶ Seizures

> **Key terms**
>
> **Hypotension** – low blood pressure.
> **Syncope** – fainting.
> **Tachycardia** – fast heart beat above 100 bpm.

The symptoms of heat exhaustion are mainly due to dehydration and an imbalance of the body's chemicals.

Heat stroke can be split into non-exertional heat stroke and exertional heat stroke.

Non-exertional heat stroke

This is caused by high external environmental temperature. Elderly people, very young children or people who are ill are more likely to become affected as they are unable to control their body temperature adequately.

Exertional heat stroke

This is brought on by physical exercise, e.g. running races or manual work, and is exacerbated by local environmental conditions. Heat stroke is a life-threatening condition that needs prompt medical intervention.

Management of hyperthermia | 8 Steps

1 Remove the casualty from the hot environment to an air-conditioned room or vehicle if possible and place them in a position they find comfortable, removing all clothing as far as possible. If you have access to a fan, this will help to cool them down, as will a wet sheet placed over them. If they are feeling dizzy, lay them down and raise their legs.

2 For casualties who present with heat stroke, facilitate cooling with cold or iced water (with some massage of the skin to ensure blood continues to flow to the surface). The application of ice packs to the casualty's neck, groin and sides of torso is also effective but wrap these up in a thin cloth first to avoid any cold injury to the skin.

3 Check the casualty's blood sugar levels if possible and manage accordingly.

4 Summon assistance at the earliest opportunity.

5 Administer oxygen as per the guidelines.

6 Complete a full set of observations and a thorough casualty assessment.

7 Record all of your findings and management on the PRF.

8 Hand the casualty over as required to the next echelon of pre-hospital care.

Cold injuries

Frostbite

Frostbite is caused when the skin becomes damaged following exposure to freezing temperatures. It most commonly affects the extremities of the body, e.g. toes, fingers, nose, ears and face.

The following table shows the three stages of frostbite.

> **Quick check**
>
> What are the signs and symptoms for a casualty with mild hypothermia?

▶ **Table 3.5**

Frostnip	Superficial frostbite	Severe frostbite
Affected area is: ▶ pale ▶ feels cold ▶ tingles ▶ numb	▶ Ice crystals may form on the skin If the casualty is back in a warm environment and their skin is being warmed they may experience: ▶ redness ▶ blisters ▶ a burning feeling ▶ swelling ▶ itching ▶ mottled skin ▶ blue or purple skin	▶ This is now affecting all the layers of the skin and the structures beneath ▶ Large blisters ▶ Skin turns black ▶ Skin feels hard to touch

Management of frostbite

7 Steps

1 Consider if the casualty is also hypothermic and manage accordingly.

2 The area needs to be rewarmed; you will need assistance from a healthcare professional as, during rewarming, the casualty will experience pain, so analgesia will be required and some of the area may need to be removed.

3 Keep the area clean and do not allow to refreeze.

4 Check for any signs of infection and manage accordingly.

5 Complete a full set of observations and a thorough casualty assessment.

6 Record all of your findings and management on the PRF.

7 Hand the casualty over as required to the next echelon of pre-hospital care.

Chilblains

Chilblains are caused by small, painful, itchy swellings of the small blood vessels in the skin. It occurs when you are repeatedly exposed to the cold and then warmed quickly. This causes a redness or dark blue colour to the area with a burning and itching sensation that becomes worse when you warm up the area. The skin becomes delicate and can break or blisters can form. There is a risk of infection if the skin breaks, so ensure it is kept clean.

Management of chilblains

6 Steps

1 Consider if the casualty is also hypothermic and manage accordingly.

2 Avoid rapid rewarming of the area.

3 Check for any signs of infection and manage accordingly.

4 Complete a full set of observations and a thorough casualty assessment.

5 Record all of your findings on the PRF.

6 Hand the casualty over as required to the next echelon of pre-hospital care.

Trenchfoot

It is thought that poor circulation combined with cold, damp conditions contributes to the development of trenchfoot. It can affect the toes, heels or the whole foot. The foot may develop: tingling, itching, pain, swelling, smell, red patches, prickly feeling, blistering and peeling skin. There is a risk of infection as open wounds develop.

Management of trenchfoot	**6 Steps**

1 Consider if the casualty is also hypothermic and manage accordingly.

2 Remove footwear; clean and dry the foot.

3 Gradually warm the feet and keep them dry. If there is any blackening to the skin, this requires immediate medical attention. Check for any signs of infection and manage accordingly.

4 Complete a full set of observations and a thorough casualty assessment.

5 Record all of your findings and management on the PRF.

6 Hand the casualty over as required to the next echelon of pre-hospital care.

Extremes of temperature in austere environments

An austere environment is an area that regularly experiences significant environmental hazards, e.g. heat, cold, and distance from definitive care, presenting you with very specific challenges when performing your role. These challenges will differ depending on the nature of the environment, so rigorous planning and preparation should be undertaken to help you understand and overcome these prior to beginning your management of the situation. You should consider the:

▶ need for shelter

▶ prolonged care of the casualty required due to an increased time for other resources to arrive

▶ need for extraction

▶ methods of extrication available including stretcher carry, air evacuation and the possible need to call specialist teams such as mountain rescue

▶ equipment you have at your disposal

▶ stretcher selection considering the terrain you will need to cover, how far you will need to go to get to a point where you can be collected by an aircraft or other vehicle, and how many people you have available to assist with moving the casualty.

> **Quick check**
>
> How would you recognise the onset of frostbite?

Understand the recognition and management of the conscious near drowned casualty

Near drowning

Link

See Unit 2, page 70 for more information on Basic Life Support.

This occurs when a casualty has been submersed for a period of time and has been unable to breathe. This causes hypoxia and can lead to death if prompt rescue, by either the casualty or others, is not achieved. There is also a risk of hypothermia and this should be considered following the rescue of any casualty who has been in water. The history leading up to the event will make these casualties easy to identify. They may:

▸ be short of breath

▸ have reduced SpO_2

▸ be fatigued

▸ have reduced level of consciousness

▸ experience respiratory and cardiac arrest.

Link

See Unit 2, page 42, for more information on ABC.

A casualty may experience these symptoms for up to 72 hours following a near drowning experience; this is often referred to as secondary drowning.

Management of near drowning   **9 Steps**

1 Manage the casualty's ABC problems first.

2 Summon assistance at the earliest opportunity.

3 There is an increased chance of the casualty vomiting, so keep this in mind when managing them.
- This is particularly important if the casualty is unable to clear their own airway.

4 If the casualty is being recovered from the water, try to remove them in a supine position.
- Avoid positioning them vertically as this can cause a sudden drop in the casualty's blood pressure. This is called hydrostatic squeeze, where the pressure of the water on the limbs increases blood pressure. When you remove this squeezing effect on the body, the blood travels back to the limbs and blood pressure drops. This can cause a loss of consciousness and in some circumstances cardiac arrest.

continued on page 119

Management of near drowning (*continued*)

5 Administer oxygen as per the guidelines.

6 Assess for, and manage, any hypothermia.

7 Complete a full set of observations and a thorough casualty assessment.

8 Record all of your findings and management on the PRF.

9 Hand the casualty over as required to the next echelon of pre-hospital care.

Assessment practice 3.3   (EC) 3.1

1 What are the signs and symptoms for a casualty who is suffering from the effects of a near drowning?

Understand the recognition and management of casualties with musculoskeletal injuries

The musculoskeletal system is a collection of bones, muscles, ligaments, tendons and other connective tissue that gives the body its form. It provides stability, protection and movement in the body.

Terminology and structure

To be able to describe any musculoskeletal injuries accurately you need to be able to identify some of the main bones and muscles in the body, plus have an understanding of some directional terms.

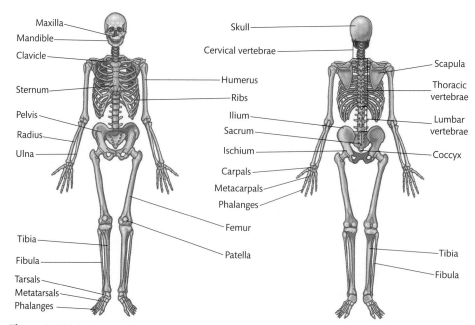

Figure 3.7 Main bones of the skeleton

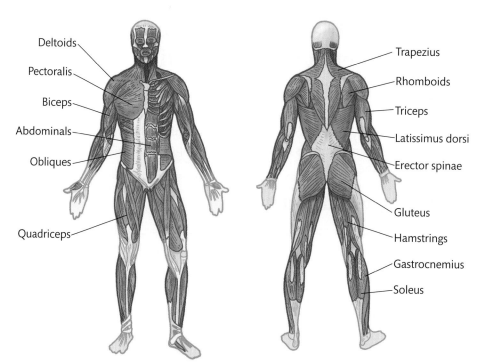

Figure 3.8 Muscles, ligaments and tendons

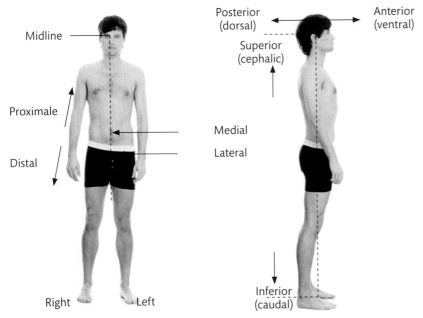

Figure 3.9 Directional terms

Fractures and dislocations

Types of fracture

Fractured bones can present in two different ways: closed or open.

Closed fracture: when the bone has broken but has not pierced the skin.

Open fracture: when the fractured bone has broken through the skin and has created an open wound. The bone may be visible as it protrudes from the open wound. In fractures that are open there is an increased risk of infection (as with any open wound), so the area should be kept as clean as possible. There may also be some active bleeding and this will need to be managed accordingly.

Dislocations

Dislocations occur in joints within the body. These can become displaced if enough force is applied in a particular direction. As a first responder it is difficult to differentiate dislocations from fractures. The management of both is the same, so there is no need for you to be able to identify if the casualty has a fracture or a dislocation, just that one of them is possible. It is possible that the casualty has both at the same site of injury.

The following table shows the signs and symptoms of a fracture or dislocation.

▶ **Table 3.6**

Signs	Symptoms
▶ Swelling	▶ Pain
▶ Bruising	▶ Reduced sensation
▶ Deformity	▶ Lack of movement
▶ **Crepitus**	▶ Tenderness
▶ Irregularities and unnatural movement	

The casualty will not necessarily present with all of these signs and symptoms, but the history of events leading up to the incident will help you decide whether they have a fracture or dislocation.

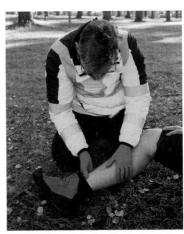

Examine the limb for a dislocation or fracture

Link

For more information on the management of bleeding, see page 139.

Key term

Crepitus – a grinding sound made by two ends of the bone rubbing together.

Quick tip

Do not try to replicate crepitus when examining a casualty.

Some fractures or dislocations have their own specific signs and symptoms to help you identify a possible injury.

▶ Neck of femur (hip): the fractured leg may be shorter than the other and externally rotated.

▶ Dislocated shoulder: the affected shoulder will look lower than the other.

Management of a closed fracture or dislocation

9 Steps

1 Manage the casualty's ABC problems first.

2 Summon assistance at the earliest opportunity.

3 Complete a full set of observations and a thorough casualty assessment.

4 Provide supplementary oxygen as required, following guidelines.

5 The limb should be immobilised.
- Ask the casualty to keep the limb still. This will prevent pain and any further damage to the surrounding tissues.
- The casualty should be placed in a position they find comfortable, supporting the affected area.
- You can help the casualty to support the limb by offering support to stabilise with your hands.
- Use an appropriate sling or splint to continue this support and immobilisation.

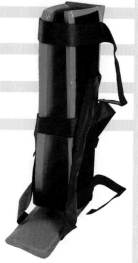
A box splint

6 Rest the limb and apply ice.
- Do not apply the ice directly to the skin but instead wrap it in a towel or similar. This helps to control swelling while not damaging the skin.

7 Document your findings relating to the limb prior to your intervention and again after any procedures.

8 Record all of your findings and management on the PRF.

9 Hand the casualty over as required to the next echelon of pre-hospital care.

Management of an open fracture

9 Steps

1 Manage the casualty's ABC problems first.

2 Summon assistance at the earliest opportunity.

3 Provide supplementary oxygen as required, following guidelines.

continued on page 123

Management of an open fracture (*continued*)

4 Control the haemorrhage as appropriate to the severity of the open wound. Do not put pressure on the exposed bone.
  - Follow haemorrhage control guidelines, keeping the wound clean to avoid infection.

5 Immobilise the limb.
  - Ask the casualty to keep the limb still. This will prevent pain and any further damage to the surrounding tissues.
  - Place the casualty in a position they find comfortable, supporting the affected area.
  - You can help the casualty to support the limb by offering support to stabilise with your hands.
  - Use an appropriate sling or splint to continue this support and immobilisation.
  - Rest the limb and apply ice.
  - Do not apply the ice directly to the skin but instead wrap it in a towel or similar. This helps to control swelling while not damaging the skin.

6 Complete a full set of observations and a thorough casualty assessment.

7 Document your findings relating to the limb prior to your intervention and again after any procedures.

8 Record all of your findings and management on the PRF.

9 Hand the casualty over as required to the next echelon of pre-hospital care.

Soft tissue injuries

Soft tissue injuries are damage caused to muscles, ligaments or tendons, normally following a sprain, strain or localised force to an area causing bruising.

These injuries can be difficult to differentiate from a fracture or dislocation and can require an x-ray at hospital to be able to diagnose the extent of the injury accurately.

A sprain is movement of an area such as a joint beyond its normal range, resulting from the stretching or tearing of ligaments. This is commonly seen in ankles, knees and wrists.

A strain is the stretching or tearing of muscles or tendons and is commonly seen in the upper leg.

Direct force applied to an area can cause bruising, which is the pooling of blood under the skin following the damage caused by the blow.

Link

See Unit 2, page 45, for more information on controlling catastrophic haemorrhage.

Management of soft tissue injuries

9 Steps

1 Manage the casualty's ABC problems first.

2 Summon assistance at the earliest opportunity if required.

3 Complete a full set of observations and a thorough casualty assessment.

continued on page 124

Management of soft tissue injuries (*continued*)

4 Provide supplementary oxygen as required following guidelines.

5 Where there is any doubt between a soft tissue injury and a fracture, the injury should be treated as a fracture.

6 For less severe soft tissue injuries:
- Place the casualty in a position they find comfortable, supporting the affected area.
- Use an appropriate sling or splint to continue this support and immobilisation.
- Rest the limb and apply ice.
- Do not apply the ice directly to the skin but instead wrap it in a towel or similar. This helps to control swelling while not damaging the skin.
- Elevate the limb to assist in swelling reduction.

The casualty may be able to walk or use the limb as normal and this is acceptable if it does not cause them pain.

7 Document your findings relating to the limb prior to your intervention and again after any procedures.

8 Record all of your findings and management on the PRF.

9 Hand the casualty over as required to the next echelon of pre-hospital care.

Pelvic fractures

Major pelvic injuries are normally seen when there is significant force involved. Therefore, in situations in which there is a significant mechanism of injury you should consider the likelihood of a pelvic fracture. For example:

- falls from height
- road traffic accidents
- crush injuries.

Pelvic fractures can be described as stable or unstable, with unstable being the more serious injury, accounting for 20 per cent of all pelvic fractures. Due to its proximity to major blood vessels, a pelvic fracture can be serious as there is the possibility of hypovolaemia and then death due to major blood loss.

Signs and symptoms of a casualty with a pelvic injury include bruising, bleeding, deformity, pain and swelling to the pelvis. Where casualties have another painful injury, such as a fractured femur, they may not describe pain in their pelvis.

> **Link**
>
> For more information on oxygen saturation, see Unit 2, page 97.

Casualties who have the possibility for major pelvic injury with major blood loss should be managed with a pelvic binder, and any movement of the casualty should be minimal and carried out carefully and in a controlled manner as these casualties are time critical. Where possible, the pelvic binder should be applied to bare skin. However, this may not be appropriate if the casualty is outside and there is a risk of hypothermia or lack of privacy. Provide supplementary oxygen as required, following guidelines.

Application of a pelvic binder

A pelvic binder should be applied in accordance with the device's instructions. The centre of the binder should be placed over the **greater trochanter**.

Key term

Greater trochanter – an anatomical part of the femur connecting to the hip bone; felt on the outside of the upper part of the leg, slightly lower than the iliac crest of the pelvis.

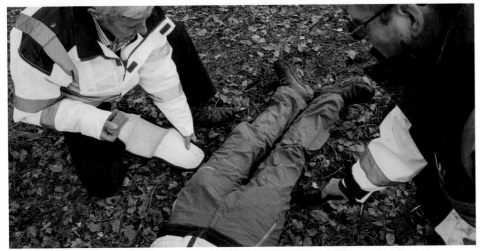

1 Place the binder under the casualty, using the natural hollows underneath them

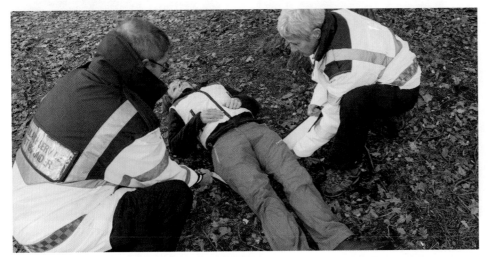

2 Use a see-saw motion to position the binder in the correct place under the casualty

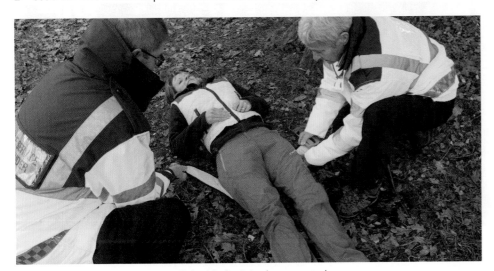

3 Continue with this motion until the binder is in the correct place

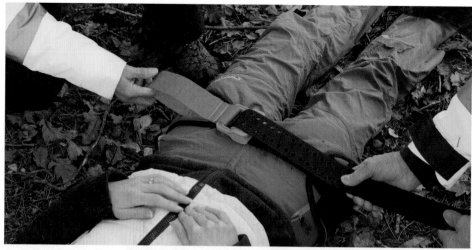

4 Fasten the pelvic binder around the casualty and tighten

Splinting, support and immobilisation

Application of a support sling

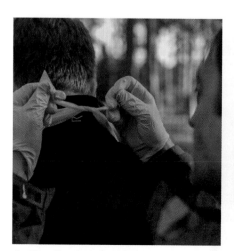

1 Place the casualty's arm across their chest

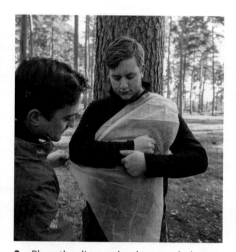

2 Place the sling under the casualty's arm

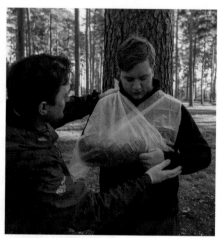

3 Take the sling over the arm to the neck

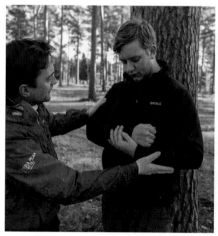

4 The sling is tied at the back of the neck

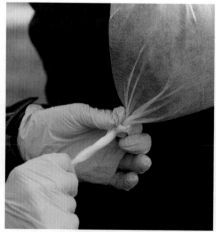

5 The sling is twisted and secured at the elbow

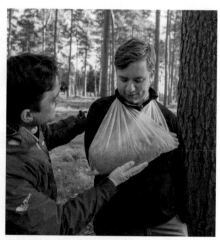

6 The completed sling

Application of an elevation sling

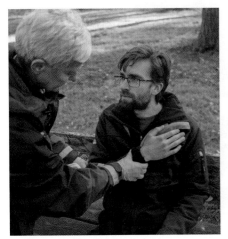

1 Place the casualty's arm high across their chest

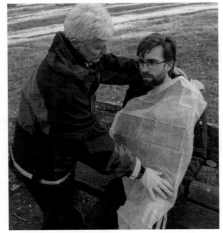

2 Place the sling over the top of the casualty's arm

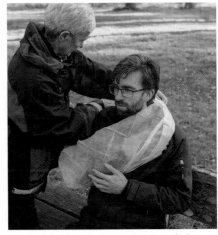

3 Take the sling around the casualty's elbow to the back

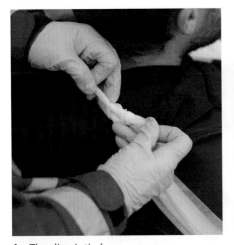

4 The sling is tied

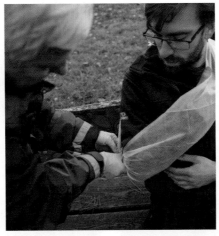

5 The sling is twisted and secured at the elbow

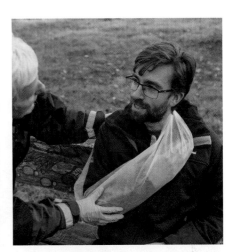

6 The completed sling

Application of a vacuum splint

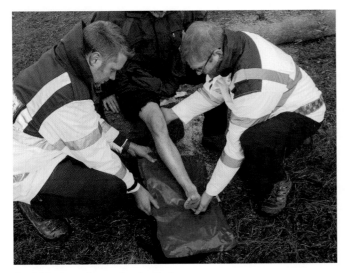

1 Slide the splint under the limb

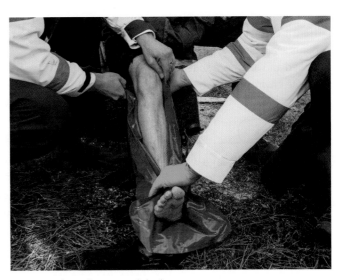

2 Wrap the splint around the leg

127

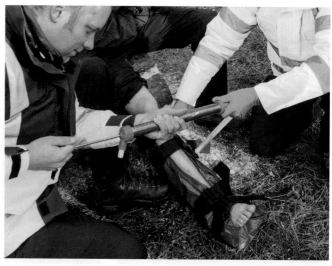

3 Fasten the splint with the straps

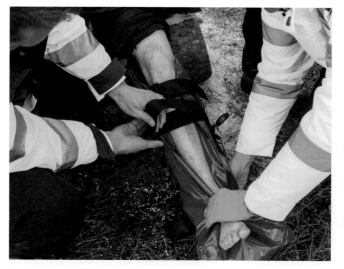

4 Use the pump to remove the air and allow the splint to form around the leg

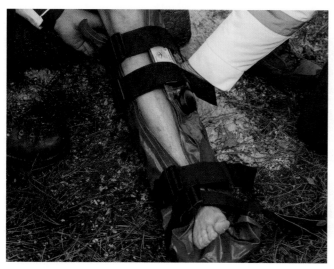

5 Splint secured

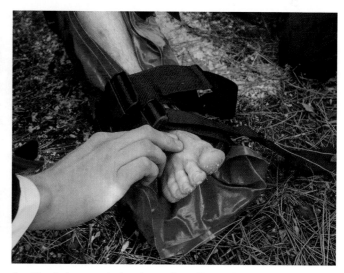

6 Check the casualty's pulse and capillary refill

Quick tip

There are other, more portable, splints available that can be applied and are more suited for remote environments.

Quick check

What type of bandage would you use when applying a support sling?

Joint and limb examinations

To be able to assess the extent of an injury you should conduct a thorough assessment of the area and document your findings. You can use the following principles when examining any potential injury.

1 Look at the limb. You may need to remove the casualty's clothes to do this.
   - Check for symmetry and swelling, using the other limb as a comparison.
   - Inspect for any bruising or wounds.

2 Feel around the area, check for swelling or deformity and compare with the other limb.
   - What is the temperature of the limb like?

3 Ask the casualty how much movement they have.
   - Is this their normal amount of movement, or is it a reduced amount or none at all?

4 Check the distal circulation.

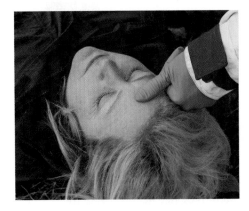 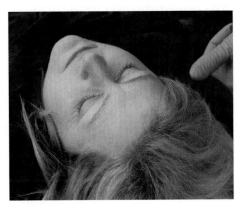

- To do this, assess the capillary refill time and look at the colour of the skin.
- You can also check a distal pulse if you are trained and competent in doing so. Compare the results with the other limb.

5 Check the sensation distal to the injury by touching both the injured and the uninjured limbs to compare.
- Ask the casualty how it feels when compared together. Is it normal? Reduced? None?

6 Check the casualty's pain. Ask them to score the pain out of 10, with 10 being the worst pain they can imagine and 0 being no pain at all. Ask them to describe the pain. Is it constant? Worse on movement? Worse on **palpation**?

Limb with compromised circulation

A limb that has a suspected fracture and signs of circulatory compromise is a limb-threatening injury and requires emergency treatment. A limb with compromised circulation will have damage to the blood supply as no oxygenated blood is making it to the tissues distal to the injury. Signs of a limb with compromised circulation are that it will:

▶ be pale

▶ have loss of movement

▶ have poor/no capillary refill

▶ have no distal pulses

▶ be cold to touch.

These limbs need to have their fractures reduced to aid circulation to the rest of the tissues. To perform this, it is recommended that the casualty has effective pain relief first, as the process of reducing the fracture is a painful one; you will need to abide by your local policy and guidelines for the administration of analgesia. Where your time for backup is greatly increased due to your location, you may have to consider performing a reduction technique prior to more senior clinical care arriving and you should follow your local policy and guidelines on this.

> **Quick check**
>
> Research the different ways in which a Structural Aluminium Malleable (SAM) splint can be used to splint an injured limb.

> **Key term**
>
> **Palpation** – touching the area.

Management of a limb with compromised circulation

8 Steps

1 Manage the casualty's ABC problems first.

2 Summon assistance at the earliest opportunity.

3 Complete a full set of observations and a thorough casualty assessment.

4 Provide supplementary oxygen as required, following guidelines.

5 For suspected compromised fractures on the shaft of the femur, apply a traction device according to the individual device instructions.

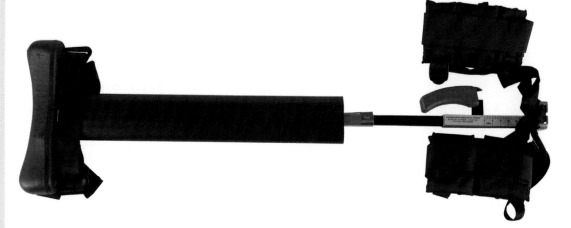

- Place the limb in traction until it is the same length as the uninjured limb. (Exercise caution if a pelvic fracture is suspected and ensure an appropriate device is selected to apply the traction.)
- For ankles with a circulatory compromise where a reduction is necessary due to the delay of more senior care, place the ankle back into **neutral alignment** by placing one hand over the top of the foot and another on the heel and pulling the foot into the correct position as if removing a wellington boot.
- Splint the limbs as appropriate.

6 Document your findings relating to the limb prior to your intervention and again after any procedures.

7 Record all of your findings and management on the PRF.

8 Hand the casualty over as required to the next echelon of pre-hospital care.

Key term

Neutral alignment – a natural position.

Assessment practice 3.4   (C) 3.2, 3.3, 3.4, 3.5, 3.8 (EC) 4.2, 4.3, 4.4, 4.5, 4.7

1 What are the signs and symptoms for a possible fracture or dislocation?

2 What is your management for a casualty suffering a suspected fracture to the upper arm?

3 What is your management of a casualty suffering a possible pelvic fracture?

Understand the recognition and management of casualties with a head injury

Mechanisms

As you are conducting your scene assessment, you should consider a possible head injury where you suspect the following mechanisms:

▶ road traffic collisions

▶ falls from standing

▶ falls from height

▶ assault

▶ falling objects

▶ contact sports.

Where a mechanism for a head injury exists you must also consider if there has been a spinal cord injury.

Minor head injury

A minor head injury can be characterised by its symptoms. It is mild and short-lived. It is often difficult in the pre-hospital environment to ascertain the seriousness of a head injury and you should always be cautious with any head injury. Signs and symptoms include:

▶ a mild headache

▶ some slightly blurred vision

▶ nausea

▶ slight dizziness

▶ small visible superficial wounds

▶ casualty is alert on AVPU.

If the casualty is taking **anticoagulants**, then they need to be assessed at hospital.

Link

See page 134 in this unit for more detail on spinal cord injuries.

Link

For more information on Alert, Voice, Pain, Unresponsive (AVPU), see Unit 2, page 43.

Key term

Anticoagulant – medication that helps prevent blood clots from forming, such as Warfarin.

Management of a minor head injury   `7 Steps`

1 Manage the casualty's ABC problems first.

2 Summon assistance if required at the earliest opportunity.

3 Complete a full set of observations and a thorough casualty assessment.

4 Manage any wounds.

5 Continue to monitor and closely observe the casualty for any signs of a serious head injury (see the following section).

continued on page 132

Management of a minor head injury (*continued*)

6 Record all of your findings and management on the PRF.

7 Hand the casualty over as required to the next echelon of pre-hospital care (if required).

Quick check

What are the signs and symptoms for a casualty who has a minor head injury?

Serious head injury

Serious head injuries can range from concussion to a more traumatic brain injury (TBI). These will have a history of a mechanism of injury that has led to the head injury being sustained. TBIs can be life-threatening injuries and the casualty may need treatment at a specialist hospital. A casualty with a serious head injury may present with some of the following signs:

▶ a reduced level of consciousness (brief or intermittent periods of consciousness)

▶ a boggy mass felt on the head on palpation

▶ leaking cerebrospinal fluid from the nose or ears

▶ vomiting

▶ hearing loss

▶ double vision

▶ difficulty staying, or keeping, awake

▶ bleeding from the ears

▶ bruising seen either behind the ears or around the eye sockets

▶ anything penetrating the head

▶ slurred or slow speech

▶ confusion

▶ a lack of coordination (ataxia)

▶ inability to walk/poor balance

▶ loss of power or sensation in limbs

▶ memory loss (amnesia)

▶ seizures or fitting

▶ significant blurred vision

▶ severe headache

▶ behaving out of character

▶ abnormal pupil reaction.

Management of a serious head injury

`9 Steps`

1 Manage the casualty's ABC problems first.

2 Summon assistance at the earliest opportunity.

continued on page 133

Management of a serious head injury (*continued*)

3 Complete a full set of observations and a thorough casualty assessment. Ensure you continually assess their consciousness level. Include a pupil reaction check using a pen torch.

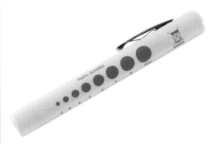
A pen torch

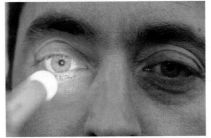
Use a pen torch to assess pupil reaction

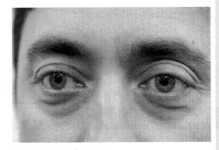
Normal pupil reaction

4 Provide supplementary oxygen as required, following guidelines.

5 Manage any wounds.

6 Consider the possibility of a spinal cord injury and manage accordingly.

7 Continue to monitor and closely observe the casualty and manage any changes. Pay particular attention to their level of consciousness.

8 Record all of your findings and management on the PRF.

9 Hand the casualty over as required to the next echelon of pre-hospital care.

Assessment practice 3.5   (C) 4.1, 4.2, 4.5 (EC) 5.1, 5.2, 5.5

1   Describe the signs and symptoms for a minor head injury?

2   What mechanisms may result in a head injury?

3   What is your management of a casualty suffering from a serious head injury?

Explore the recognition and management of a casualty with a spinal injury

The spine is a structure in the back made up of irregularly shaped bones called vertebrae. These bones are divided up into areas of the column and given a number for identification.

These are:

▸ Cervical spine: 7 vertebrae (C1–C7)

▸ Thoracic spine: 12 vertebrae (T1–T12)

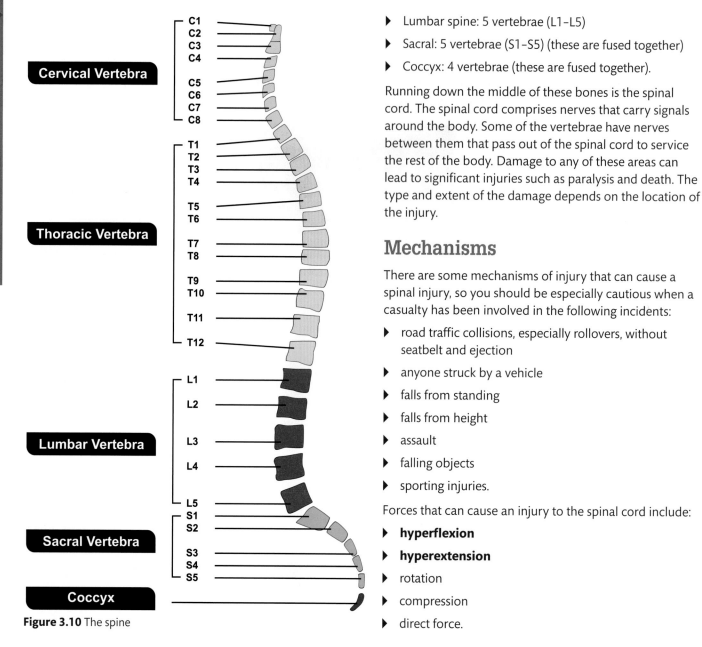

Cervical Vertebra
- C1
- C2
- C3
- C4
- C5
- C6
- C7
- C8

Thoracic Vertebra
- T1
- T2
- T3
- T4
- T5
- T6
- T7
- T8
- T9
- T10
- T11
- T12

Lumbar Vertebra
- L1
- L2
- L3
- L4
- L5

Sacral Vertebra
- S1
- S2
- S3
- S4
- S5

Coccyx

Figure 3.10 The spine

▶ Lumbar spine: 5 vertebrae (L1–L5)

▶ Sacral: 5 vertebrae (S1–S5) (these are fused together)

▶ Coccyx: 4 vertebrae (these are fused together).

Running down the middle of these bones is the spinal cord. The spinal cord comprises nerves that carry signals around the body. Some of the vertebrae have nerves between them that pass out of the spinal cord to service the rest of the body. Damage to any of these areas can lead to significant injuries such as paralysis and death. The type and extent of the damage depends on the location of the injury.

Mechanisms

There are some mechanisms of injury that can cause a spinal injury, so you should be especially cautious when a casualty has been involved in the following incidents:

▶ road traffic collisions, especially rollovers, without seatbelt and ejection

▶ anyone struck by a vehicle

▶ falls from standing

▶ falls from height

▶ assault

▶ falling objects

▶ sporting injuries.

Forces that can cause an injury to the spinal cord include:

▶ **hyperflexion**

▶ **hyperextension**

▶ rotation

▶ compression

▶ direct force.

Key terms

Hyperflexion – where the head is forced forwards so the chin moves towards the chest.

Hyperextension – where the head is forced backwards so the rear of the head moves towards the base of the neck.

Specific symptoms of a spinal cord injury

The casualty may experience some of the following:

▶ pain in the neck

▶ pain in the back

▶ tingling, numbness or a burning sensation in the limbs or trunk

▶ loss or reduction in sensation in the limbs

▶ loss or reduction of movement in the limbs

▶ sharp shooting pains

▶ loss of bladder or bowel control.

In the unconscious trauma casualty or where there has been a significant mechanism, always presume a spinal cord injury and manage appropriately.

Management of a spinal cord injury

9 Steps

1 Apply manual in-line stabilisation (MILS) (see the following section) as soon as possible to any casualty who you suspect has a spinal cord injury. Also tell them to keep as still as they can.

2 Manage the casualty's ABC problems.

3 Summon assistance at the earliest opportunity.

4 Complete a full set of observations and a thorough casualty assessment.

5 Provide supplementary oxygen as required following guidelines.

6 Communication with the casualty is vital to make sure they know what and why you are applying these techniques; this will also help keep them still.

7 Vomiting carries a specific risk at this point as once they are immobilised they will be unable to clear their airway.
  • You must have a plan should the casualty begin to vomit: this may include 'log rolling' the casualty onto their side while maintaining MILS.

8 Where immobilisation is required, there are only two methods of providing this: (a) MILS with the back supported and (b) collar, head blocks and back support.

9 Continue to monitor and closely observe the casualty and manage any changes. Record all of your findings and management on the PRF. Hand over the casualty as required to the next echelon of pre-hospital care.

Manual in-line stabilisation (MILS)

Talk to the casualty and ask them to keep their head still. Place your hands either side of the casualty's head and keep the head secure. The centre of the face should run down the centre of the chest.

Removal of a helmet

You may come across a casualty who is wearing a helmet such as a motorcycle helmet, bike helmet or climbing helmet. You may suspect a spinal cord injury in these cases.

There may be times when you need to remove a casualty's helmet to enable management of the casualty. This may be required if:

▶ there is a problem with the casualty's airway or you are unable to assess it

▶ you need better access to provide any breaths required if the casualty is in arrest

▶ you need to immobilise the casualty using head blocks and the helmet is preventing this

▶ you need to immobilise the casualty using a cervical collar and the helmet is preventing this

▶ you need to assess the head more thoroughly.

Quick check

What are the signs and symptoms of a casualty who may have suffered a spinal injury?

The speed with which you perform the removal will depend upon the reasons you need access. If a situation is life threatening, the helmet may need to be removed quickly and carefully. If the situation is not life threatening and removing the helmet would exacerbate the symptoms, then do not remove the helmet and wait until more qualified help arrives.

To remove the helmet in a safe and controlled manner requires two people. If the situation is life threatening, this may not always be possible if you do not have the resources.

Removal of a helmet

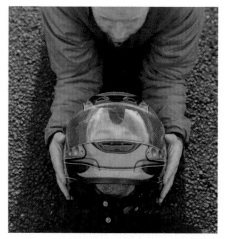

1 One responder holds the casualty's head in line with his body

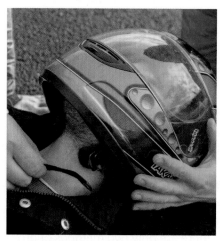

2 One responder holds the casualty's head while the other unfastens the helmet's chin strap

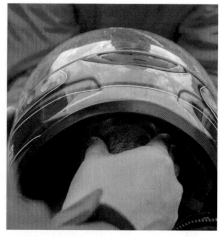

3 Still holding the head still, position the hand as shown

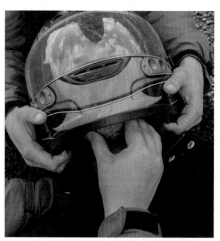

4 One responder keeps the head still while the other changes the grip on the helmet

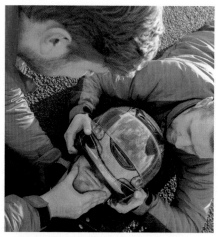

5 Rock the helmet backwards while pulling it outward from each side

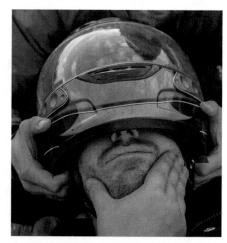

6 One responder rocks the helmet forwards while the other keeps the head still

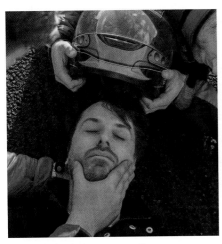

7 With the helmet now off, one responder takes control of the casualty's head

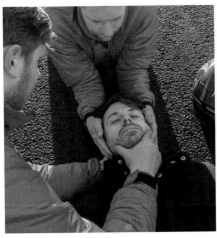

8 One responder keeps the head still while the other cushions it

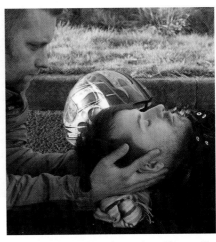

9 With the head cushioned and kept still, await further support

Application of rigid cervical collar

Rigid cervical collars can be used in the stabilisation of a casualty's cervical spine during extrication. Exercise caution if the casualty also has a head injury as this can increase **intracranial pressure**. Some casualties dislike collars as they find them uncomfortable or restrictive to their breathing. Take a 'best possible' approach in these cases.

> **Key term**
>
> **Intracranial pressure** – the pressure inside the skull and therefore in the brain tissue and cerebrospinal fluid.

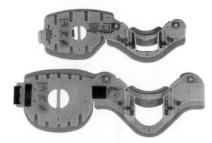

Cervical collars come in different sizes

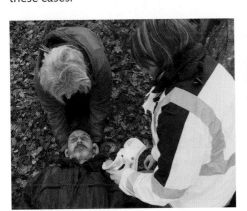

1 Prepare to apply the cervical collar on the casualty. Two responders are required.

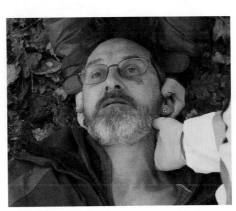

2 Measure the casualty for the correct collar size

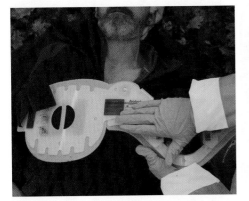

3 Adjust the collar to the correct size

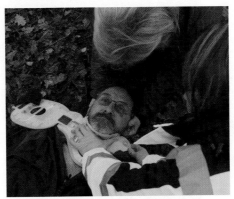

4 Place the collar on the front of the casualty and ensure the chin and chest piece is central

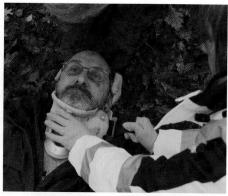

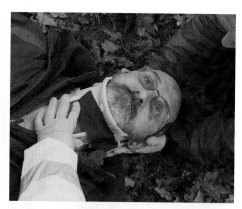

5 Feed the back of the collar around the casualty's neck while holding the front in place

6 Secure the fastening strap at the front of the collar

Packaging of the casualty

The orthopaedic scoop stretcher is ergonomically designed and can be split into two halves to allow for minimal movement of the casualty while packaging.

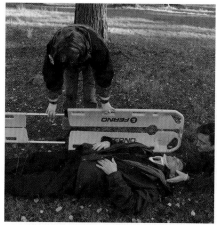

1 Measure the scoop against the size of the casualty and adjust accordingly

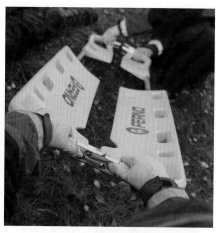

2 Separate the scoop into two halves

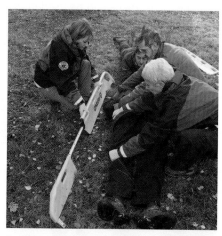

3 Roll the casualty a small amount towards the team, moving together and keeping the head and neck in neutral alignment: slide the first half of the stretcher underneath the casualty

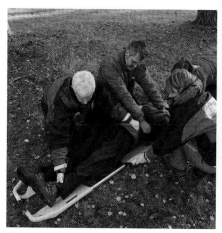

4 Repeat this on the other side

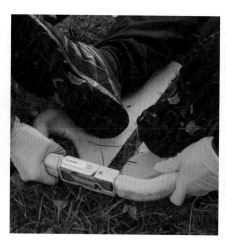

5 Click the stretcher halves together

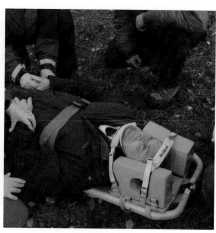

6 Use straps to immobilise the body and head blocks to immobilise the head

The vacuum mattress is a device into which the casualty is placed. Removing the air allows the mattress to form around the casualty's body into a hard, immobilising device. The casualty is best placed on this using an orthopaedic scoop stretcher.

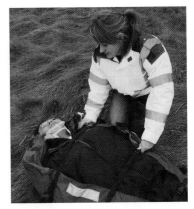

A vacuum mattress

Assessment practice 3.6	(C) 5.2, 5.3 (EC) 6.2, 6.3

1 What are the signs and symptoms for a possible spinal injury?

2 What is your management for a casualty suffering a suspected spinal injury?

Understand the recognition and management of casualties with wounds and bleeding

Wound types

Wounds have different characteristics depending upon their cause.

▸ blunt, e.g. bruising, grazes, **avulsion**

▸ penetrating, e.g. gunshots, cuts with a sharp object, having an object embedded within them

▸ blast, e.g. caused following an explosion.

Management of non-catastrophic bleeding

Haemorrhages are either compressible or non-compressible.

▸ Compressible injuries are located on the limbs and can be controlled easily using pressure and, where required, the application of a tourniquet.

▸ Non-compressible wounds are more difficult to manage as a tourniquet cannot be applied and this may require drug administration or surgery in the pre-hospital or hospital environment to stop the active bleeding.

Non-catastrophic haemorrhaging

Controlling blood loss:

1 Apply a dressing.

2 Apply lots of direct pressure directly over the wound.

3 Where possible, elevate the wound above the heart.

If bleeding is not controlled:

1 Apply further dressings.

2 Continue to apply direct pressure.

If bleeding is still not under control, then treat this as a catastrophic haemorrhage.

> **Key term**
>
> **Avulsion** – where the skin is torn from the tissues (also known as degloving).

> **Link**
>
> See Unit 2, page 45 for catastrophic haemorrhage management.

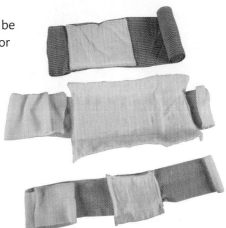

A selection of dressing types

Applying a dressing

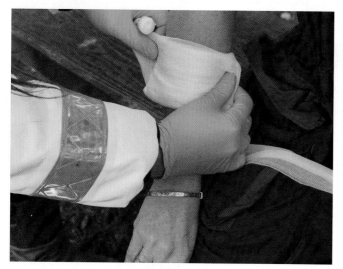

1 Place the absorbant pad over the wound

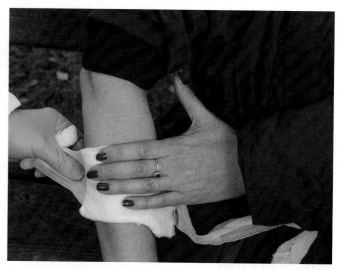

2 Ask the casualty to place their other hand over the wound to maintain the pressure

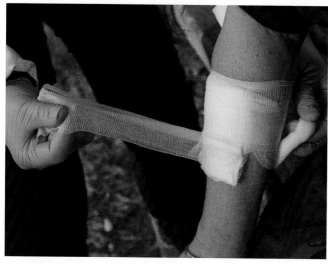

3 Wrap the bandage around the arm, sealing both sides of the absorbant pad

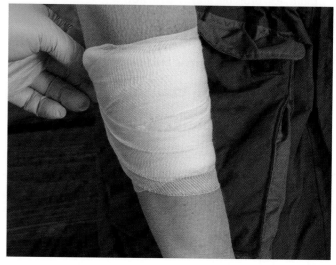

4 Completion of the dressing

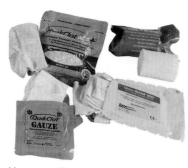

Haemostatic gauzes

Haemostatics

Haemostatic gauze can be used to assist in the stopping of bleeding. It works by promoting clotting using gauze impregnated with chemicals that are used to stop bleeding by creating a gel like plug in the wound. Open the gauze pack and feed it into the wound to pack the whole injury site and apply pressure on top. Never cut this gauze; place any spare loosely onto the surface of the skin underneath the bandage.

Splintage

Splinting injured limbs is important in helping to reduce bleeding. For femurs, place a traction device onto the injured leg to reduce the fracture and control the bleeding. Apply this following the manufacturer's instructions. See page 127 for more information on applying splints.

Internal bleeding

In addition to bleeding wounds, it is possible for the casualty to lose circulating blood volume internally into the tissues and cavities within the body.

Some of the possible areas where large volumes of blood can be lost are:

▶ chest cavity

▶ abdominal cavity

▶ pelvic cavity

▶ tissues surrounding the long bones, e.g. thigh muscle surrounding the femur.

You must be aware of the signs and symptoms of internal bleeding and ensure that you summon assistance at the earliest opportunity as, depending on where the injury is, there is little you can do to manage it. Signs and symptoms of internal bleeding may be:

▶ increased heart rate

▶ increased respiration

▶ reduced consciousness

▶ agitation

▶ bruising around the area

▶ pain

▶ pale skin

▶ dizziness

▶ nausea

▶ vomiting.

> **Quick check**
>
> Name four locations in the body from which a casualty can lose a significant amount of blood internally.

Amputations

Amputations and partial amputations are also wounds and can involve the whole, or part of, digits and limbs. They can also be classified as partial or complete. A partial amputation is where there is still some tissue, bone or muscle connecting the part to the body.

Management of amputations　　　　　　　　　　　　　**9 Steps**

1 Manage any catastrophic haemorrhage and the casualty's ABC problems.

2 Summon assistance at the earliest opportunity.

3 Complete a full set of observations and a thorough casualty assessment.

4 Provide supplementary oxygen as required, following guidelines.

5 Recover the amputated part if possible, removing any dirt from it using sterile saline.

continued on page 142

Management of amputations (*continued*)

6 Wrap the amputated part in sterile saline-soaked gauze, place it in a container or re-sealable plastic bag, and place into ice. (Do not place the amputated part directly on the ice.)

7 Continue to monitor and closely observe the casualty and manage any changes.

8 Record all of your findings and management on the PRF.

9 Hand the casualty over as required to the next echelon of pre-hospital care.

Nose bleeds

Link

See Unit 2, page 45 for more on catastrophic haemorrhage.

Nose bleeds (also known as epistaxis) can be alarming for the casualty as there is often a large amount of blood. They can be caused by a traumatic injury, such as a fall or a blunt force, and it is important to perform a full assessment to ensure there are no other injuries.

Management of nose bleeds

7 Steps

1 The casualty should be sitting down.

2 Pinch the nose at the soft part just below the bone and above the nostrils. This should be done for at least 10 minutes before letting go.

3 While this is happening it is important to tilt the head forward, not back. This helps to stop blood from passing down the back of the nose and down the throat.

4 Place some ice, wrapped in material, over the nose. This will cause the blood vessels to constrict and will help to stop the bleeding.

5 Tell the casualty to breathe via their mouth and not to inhale through their nose as this can cause the bleeding to start again.

6 If the bleeding has not stopped after 20 minutes of pinching the nose, then summon assistance via the ambulance service, or accident and emergency.

7 Monitor the casualty for hypovolaemic shock and manage accordingly.

Facial injury

Link

For more on hypovolaemia, see page 143.

If the casualty has suffered a facial injury and there is active bleeding, you must ensure their airway is clear (you may need to use suction). In a conscious casualty they should be sitting upright. In the unconscious casualty the safe airway position should be used. Monitor the casualty continuously. You should also consider the likelihood of a head and spinal injury and manage accordingly.

Crush injury

Crush injuries are a rare occurrence but should be considered in industrial accidents or road traffic collisions, for example. These casualties need expert medical attention quickly and you should summon assistance immediately. Where possible, the casualty should be released as soon as possible, irrespective of the time they have been crushed. Manage the casualty following oxygen guidelines and control any bleeding. Keep them calm and keep them warm with blankets to prevent hypothermia. Monitor the casualty closely at all times.

| Assessment practice 3.7 | (C) 6.2, 6.5 (EC) 7.2, 7.5 |

1 What are the signs and symptoms of internal blood loss?

2 What is your management for a casualty with an amputated thumb?

Understand the recognition and management of a casualty suffering from hypovolaemic shock

Hypovolaemic shock is defined as a lack of circulating blood volume leading to an inadequate perfusion of tissues with oxygen. This can be a result of blood loss following trauma or severe dehydration.

Stages of hypovolaemic shock

As a guide, the amount of fluid loss can be classified into four stages, with associated signs and symptoms. This should be viewed as a continuum and the casualty will present somewhere along this line. It is a guide based upon the percentage of blood volume lost, and the figures of actual volume are based on an average amount within an average adult.

▶ **Table 3.7**

	Stage 1	Stage 2	Stage 3	Stage 4
% of blood lost	0%–15%	15%–30%	30%–40%	40%+
Amount of blood for an average adult	0 ml–750 ml	750 ml–1500 ml	1500 ml–2000 ml	2000 ml+
Heart rate	Normal	Above 100 bpm	Above 120 bpm	Above 140 bpm
Respiration rate	Normal	Above 20	Above 30	Above 40
Mental state	Normal Slight anxiety	Anxiety Restless	Confused Agitated	Reduced level of consciousness
Skin	Pale	Pale, cool, clammy	Pale, increased **diaphoresis**	Extreme diaphoresis
Capillary refill	Normal	Delayed	Delayed	Absent

Key term

Diaphoresis – sweating.

Management of hypovolaemic shock

9 Steps

1 Manage any catastrophic haemorrhage and manage the casualty's ABC problems.

2 Summon assistance at the earliest opportunity.

3 Where possible, you must treat the cause of the hypovolaemia to stop any further bleeding.

4 Keep the casualty warm and, if their injuries allow, carefully place them on the floor and raise their legs.

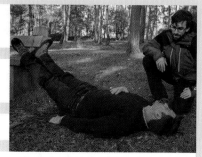

5 Assess any areas where the casualty is experiencing pain and conduct a thorough secondary survey.

6 Complete a full set of observations and a thorough secondary assessment.

7 Provide supplementary oxygen as required, following guidelines.

8 Continue to monitor and closely observe the casualty and manage any changes.

9 Record all of your findings and management on the PRF. Hand the casualty over as required to the next echelon of pre-hospital care.

Link

For more information on catastrophic haemorrhage, please see Unit 2, page 45.

Assessment practice 3.8

(C) 7.1, 7.2 (EC) 8.1, 8.2

1 Describe the stages of hypovolaemic shock. Use the text on signs and symptoms to help you.

2 What is your management for a casualty suffering from hypovolaemic shock?

Understand the recognition and management of casualties with chest injuries

The structure and contents of the thoracic cavity protect many important organs that are vital to life, such as the heart, lungs and arteries (see **Figure 3.11**). In casualties who have experienced trauma, chest injuries are one of the most common causes of death.

Injuries that can be found following a traumatic incident include:

▸ flail chest

▸ fractured ribs

▸ tension pneumothorax

▸ open chest wound

▸ massive haemothorax.

Any chest injury can adversely affect the casualty's breathing. The mechanisms involved with breathing mean that chest and diaphragm movement creates a vacuum sucking air into the lungs; as these structures return, the air is expelled. If there is damage to the chest, then the casualty may guard from any pain by changing the way in which they breathe. If there is a hole, then this vacuum may not be created and breathing will become less effective.

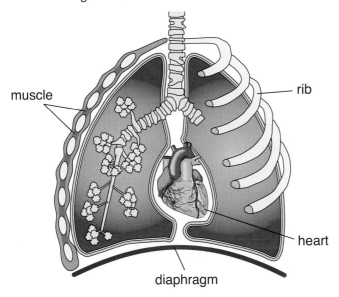

muscle

rib

heart

diaphragm

Figure 3.11 The structure and contents of the thorax

Flail segment

A flail segment is caused by blunt trauma to the chest wall. It is defined as two or more consecutive ribs fractured in two or more places. This creates a section of ribs that are no longer attached to the rest of the rib cage. This can also happen to the sternum if there are fractures to all the ribs on each side of the sternum, causing the sternum to be detached. This flail segment then moves independently with the rest of the chest during breathing, causing pain and reduced volume of breathing. You can see this unnatural movement of the flail segment when you inspect the casualty. It causes 'paradoxical movement' – when the casualty takes a breath in, the chest would normally expand, but this flail segment is sucked in. Signs and symptoms of a flail chest include:

- pain on breathing
- pain on movement
- mechanism of injury
- history
- **paradoxical breathing**

- **tachyponia** or **bradyponia**
- cyanosis
- reduced SpO_2 level
- pain on palpation
- shallow breathing.

Fractured ribs

Ribs can be fractured when a casualty falls or they experience direct blows to the chest. They can be very painful, especially when the casualty breathes in and out. Signs and symptoms of broken ribs include:

- pain on breathing in
- pain on movement
- pain on palpation

- swelling over the site of the injury
- bruising over the site of the injury
- shallow breathing.

Key terms

Paradoxical breathing – the chest moves inward during inhalation instead of outward.

Tachyponia – quick breathing.

Bradyponia – slow breathing.

Quick check

What is meant by a flail segment?

Tension pneumothorax

A tension pneumothorax can be caused by a traumatic incident or it can be spontaneous. It is a rare injury caused when the lung is damaged and results in air leaking out into the space surrounding the lung. For breathing to be effective a vacuum must be created within the thoracic cavity to suck air into the lungs. This leaked air has nowhere to go, so remains in the space between the lung and the chest. With each breath that is taken this amount of air increases. The air in the cavity causes the lung to collapse so that it does not function effectively. This creates extra pressure on the other lung and the heart. If this pressure is not released externally, then as the pressure increases the heart and lungs will be unable to function and the casualty will go into cardiac arrest. If you suspect a tension pneumothorax, you must summon assistance as soon as possible. Signs and symptoms of a tension pneumothorax include the following:

▶ reduced chest movement on the injured side

▶ injured side appears over expanded

▶ neck veins can become distended

▶ casualty's breathing gets rapidly worse

▶ casualty may experience pain and/or anxiety

▶ struggling to breathe

▶ reduced SpO_2

▶ increased respiration rate

▶ collapse/unconsciousness.

Massive haemothorax

A haemothorax is a collection of blood in the space between the lung and the chest wall. It can be caused by blunt or penetrating trauma. Small haemothoraces are self-limiting. However, if the bleeding is more severe and remains active, the pleural space will decrease and symptoms will worsen. Signs and symptoms of a haemothorax include:

▶ chest pain and/or anxiety

▶ signs of hypovolaemia

▶ difficulty breathing

▶ rapid heart rate

▶ rapid, shallow breathing

▶ restlessness

▶ shortness of breath

▶ collapse/unconsciousness.

Open chest wound

An open chest wound as a direct result of penetrating trauma is a potentially life-threatening condition and you should summon assistance at the earliest available opportunity. Seal open chest wounds with a non-occlusive dressing. These dressings allow air and fluid to escape and prevent a tension pneumothorax from forming. Where the object has penetrated and remains embedded, do not remove it. Handle this carefully and secure it with a dressing. If the object is pulsating, do not prevent this from happening. Where the casualty has one open chest wound, you must search the rest of their body for further injuries and wounds.

Place the casualty in a sitting position to ease their breathing. If the wound has been caused by a gunshot, search for an exit wound as well as an entry wound. Signs and symptoms of a casualty with an open chest wound will vary depending upon the extent of the injury but could include:

▸ signs of tension pneumothorax

▸ signs of haemothorax

▸ a visible open wound

▸ the history of events leading up to the injury

▸ pain at the site of the injury.

Conducting a chest examination

Carry out the following steps when conducting a chest examination:

R – Respiration rate

V – Volume of breathing

P – Put oxygen on now

F – Feel the chest

L – Look at the chest

A – Armpits

S – Search the back and sides

H – Holes

Respiration rate: count the casualty's respiration rate. You can do this by counting for 15 seconds then multiplying the result by 4 to give you the number of breaths they are taking in a minute. For an adult a normal rate would be between 12 and 20.

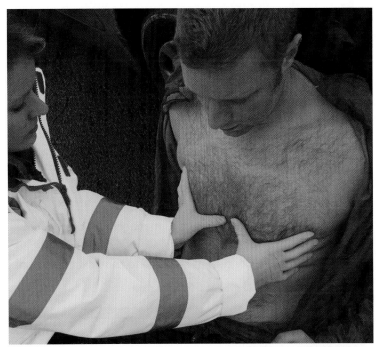

Conducting a chest examination

Volume of breathing: you need to look at what sort of depth of breath the casualty is taking. Judge this by looking at how much the chest is expanding. You can also place your hands on the bottom of the ribs to feel how much movement the chest makes on each breath. While you are doing this, you can feel if each side is expanding equally.

Put oxygen on now: administer oxygen as per the guidelines. In major trauma the addition of supplementary oxygen is indicated using a non-rebreather (reservoir) mask.

Feel the chest: as well as feeling for the chest movement, you should also feel the chest for any deformity, swelling, flailed segments and wounds. While you are feeling the chest the casualty can tell you if they experience any pain. You may wish to then focus more on any areas where they feel pain when you palpate.

Look at the chest: as well as looking for the volume as just described, you can also look at the chest to see if there are any marks that could give you an indication of any injuries. Check for bruising, swelling, redness, wounds and deformity.

Armpits: remember that the armpits also form part of the chest and these too should have the same examination as the rest.

Search the back and sides: search all around the thoracic cavity as you would the rest of the chest. This is particularly important if the casualty has a penetrating wound, as there may be more than one wound.

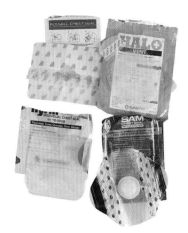

Holes: cover them with a non-occlusive dressing to allow air and fluid to drain from the wound and no air to pass back into the cavity.

Non-occlusive dressings

Management of a chest injury

9 Steps

1 Manage any catastrophic haemorrhage and the casualty's ABC problems.

2 Summon assistance at the earliest opportunity.

3 Cover any wounds with a non-occlusive dressing.

4 Provide supplementary oxygen as required, following guidelines.

5 Complete a full set of observations and a thorough casualty assessment.

6 Position the casualty where they are most comfortable.
- If there is no indication of a possible spinal injury or other injuries, ask the casualty to sit upright or lean back in a semi-recumbent position as this will allow them to breathe more easily.

7 Continue to monitor and closely observe the casualty and manage any changes.

8 Record all of your findings and management on the PRF.

9 Hand the casualty over as required to the next echelon of pre-hospital care.

Link

For more on catastrophic haemorrhage, see Unit 2, page 45.

Assessment practice 3.9   (C) 3.9 (EC) 9.1, 9.3

1 What are the signs and symptoms of a chest injury?

2 What is your management for a casualty with a suspected chest injury following a kick by a horse?

Understand the principles of manual handling and casualty extraction

There are inherent risks with any type of moving or manual handling of casualties and you should ensure you take reasonable steps to prevent injury to yourself, colleagues and the casualty. People are difficult to manoeuvre and can be heavy. The amount of handling required will vary depending on your area of operation and local policy. It is vitally important that any manual handling tasks are completed within your level of training and local policy.

Manual handling injuries

Manual handling injuries include both soft tissue injuries (sprains and strains) and skeletal injuries such as fractures.

Dynamic manual handling risk assessment

Before performing any manual handling task, you should carry out a dynamic personal risk assessment to ensure that it is safe for you and the casualty. This comprises five steps:

▶ task

▶ individual

▶ load

▶ environment

▶ other factors.

You need to ask yourself questions about each of the steps in the assessment, as shown in the table below.

▶ **Table 3.8**

Task	▶ What needs to be done? ▶ Does everyone know the plan? ▶ Is it necessary? ▶ Where do you need to go from and to? ▶ Is there any twisting involved? ▶ Do you need to do any bending? ▶ Can the distance be reduced? ▶ Is this urgent?
Individual	▶ Can the person or people conducting the task do it safely? ▶ Do you have any injuries? ▶ Is it within their capability and training? ▶ How experienced are you at this? ▶ Do you have enough people?
Load	▶ How heavy is the load? ▶ How can it be gripped? ▶ Is the weight equal? ▶ Where is the centre of gravity? ▶ Is the load stable? ▶ Is the load unpredictable?
Environment	▶ How much space do you have? Can you give yourself more space? ▶ What is the ground like? ▶ Are there any weather considerations? ▶ Are there any obstacles? ▶ Are there any steps or stairs? ▶ What is the lighting like?
Other factors	▶ Do you all have the correct Personal Protective Equipment (PPE)? ▶ Is there any equipment that would make this task safer? ▶ Ensure good, clear communication.

Quick check

When performing a manual handling task, what are the five steps to consider when assessing the risk?

Lifting

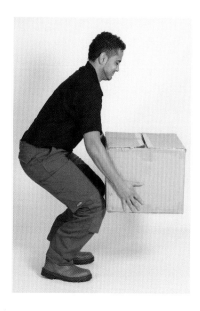

Good handling techniques for lifting are important to reduce the risk and to ensure the safety of all involved. Some practical tips adapted from the Health and Safety Executive guidance are:

▶ Think – plan the lift and use the earlier TILEO model.

▶ Adopt a stable position with your feet slightly apart and one leg slightly forward. Make sure you have the correct footwear and clothing.

▶ Get a good grip and keep the load close to the body.

▶ Start in a good posture with slight bending of the back, hips and knees.

▶ Do not flex the back any further while lifting.

▶ Keep the load close to your waist.

▶ Avoid twisting the back or leaning to the side. Shoulders and hips should be level at all times, and move your feet to turn accordingly.

▶ Keep your head up while handling.

▶ Move smoothly and do not jerk at the load.

Pushing and pulling

Some practical tips adapted from the Health and Safety Executive guidance are:

▶ Handling devices – use aids where possible. These must be well-maintained.

▶ Where possible, you should push rather than pull.

▶ Do not attempt to negotiate slopes or ramps on your own. You should have another colleague to help you.

▶ Moving an object over an uneven or soft surface requires additional force.

▶ Keep feet well away from the load and go no faster than walking pace.

Manual handling in cardiorespiratory arrest

Where the casualty is in cardiac or respiratory arrest, there are different ways in which you can transfer the casualty to the floor to begin your management. Which technique you will use will depend on the number of trained people available.

One-person technique

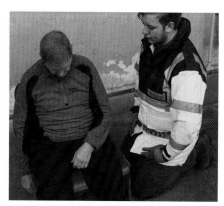

1 Kneel on the floor to the side of the casualty

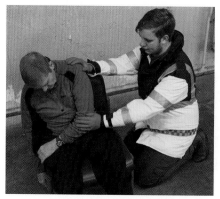

2 Position the casualty's arm that is closest to you across their body and push them away from you

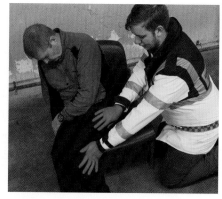

3 Push against the casualty's lower thigh with both hands

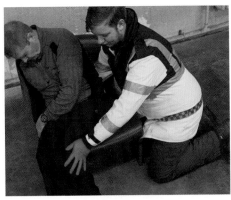

4 Place one hand behind the casualty to try and reach their opposite hip

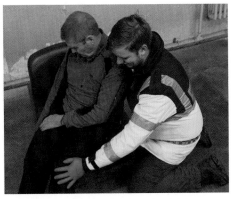

5 Place your other hand on the thigh closest to you

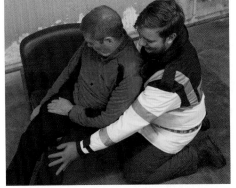

6 Pull with your hand at the back and push with your hand on the thigh to move the casualty to the floor

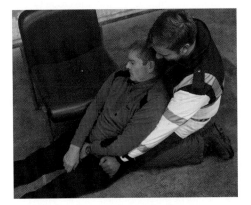

7 Position the casualty on the floor

Two-person technique

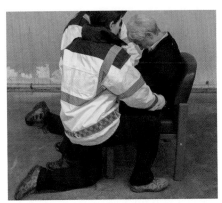

1 Kneel on the floor in front of, and slightly to the side of, the casualty's chair

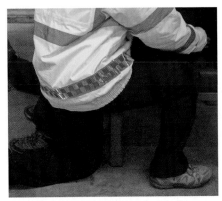

2 Your innermost knee should be on the floor and outermost knee should be bent upwards with your foot flat on the floor

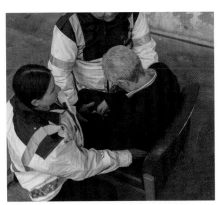

3 With your outermost hand take hold of the casualty's lower back in the hip area and your innermost hand under the casualty's knee

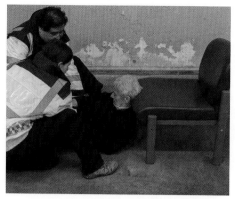 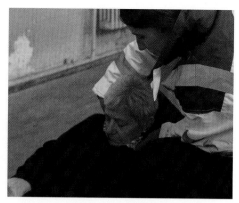

4 Under the direction of one responder, sit back towards your ankle using your body weight; this will pull the casualty forward and onto the floor

5 Position the casualty away from the chair using their legs, while the second responder supports the head

Where a third responder is available, they can support the casualty's head as they are moved to the floor.

Importance of manual handling techniques

Good manual handing techniques are important for both you and the casualty.

▶ **Table 3.9**

Benefits to the casualty	Benefits to the first responder
▶ Reduces the risk of their condition worsening ▶ Helps to maintain dignity	▶ Helps to reduce the risk of injury ▶ Reduces the risk of any injury having an impact on your ability to undertake work ▶ Any injury will impact on your ability to complete tasks and impact on your leisure time ▶ Preservation of your fitness level both now and in later life ▶ Reduces the risk of litigation for the first responder and their employer

Use of stretchers

There are many different types of stretchers available, each with their own advantages and disadvantages in different situations and for different casualties.

Some examples of the different types of stretcher available include:

▶ orthopaedic scoop stretcher

▶ semi-rigid, e.g. a Multi-integrated Body Splint Stretcher (MIBS)

▶ rigid, e.g. basket stretcher.

▶ **Table 3.10**

Orthopaedic scoop stretcher: Useful when immobilising casualties if you suspect a spinal injury, as it ensures there is minimal movement, e.g. in trauma casualties.

Advantages	Disadvantages	
▶ No or minimal movement needed when immobilising a possible spinal injury ▶ Can be split into two ▶ Can get casualties off the floor with minimal movement ▶ Reduced manual handling from the rescuer to get the casualty onto the stretcher when immobile or with a reduced consciousness ▶ Can fold in half for easy storage ▶ Can be used with head blocks for spinal immobilisation ▶ Adjustable in length ▶ Firm ▶ Light ▶ X-ray translucent ▶ Plastic and easy to clean ▶ Can be used to move a casualty into another stretcher if required	▶ Hard to carry a casualty for long distances due to its slim design ▶ Does not collapse small for moving to a casualty ▶ Cannot be used in conjunction with rope systems for lowering or lifting the casualty during a rescue ▶ There is a weight limit that can vary depending on the manufacture but is lower than other types of stretchers	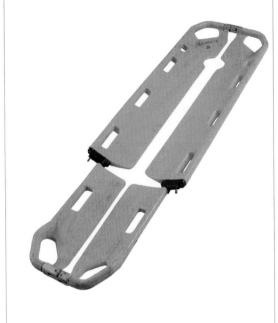

▶ **Table 3.11**

MIBS stretcher: Useful when in a confined space during a rescue or technical rescue when mobility of the stretcher is important.

Advantages	Disadvantages	
▶ Small when packed away ▶ Easily carried to the casualty ▶ Light ▶ Accessories to customise the stretcher for your needs ▶ Narrow form ▶ Handles for the rescuer ▶ Insulation to keep the casualty warm ▶ Can be used for technical rescue ▶ Can be dragged	▶ Made from fabric, so bodily fluids can become absorbed, making it unusable ▶ Hard to clean ▶ Can be difficult to accommodate larger casualties	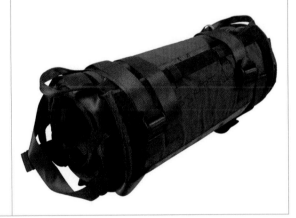

▶ **Table 3.12**

Basket stretcher: Useful if protection from the ground for the casualty is needed, for long-distance extrication or technical rescue, or if it needs to be mounted onto other devices.

Advantages	Disadvantages	
▶ Strong, rigid design ▶ Can be used for technical rope rescue ▶ Can be used to slide the casualty along the ground in some conditions ▶ Foam padding to provide comfort and to reduce pressure areas ▶ Some stretchers will fold in half for transport and storage ▶ Lots of handling points ▶ Can be carried by multiple people over a long distance ▶ Can attach devices such as wheels and straps to the stretcher to allow for long-distance extrications ▶ Can be used for helicopter winching	▶ Requires other stretchers to be used for spinal immobilisation ▶ Large size – some of these are designed to be split in two for ease of storage and for carrying to the casualty but they are still bulky	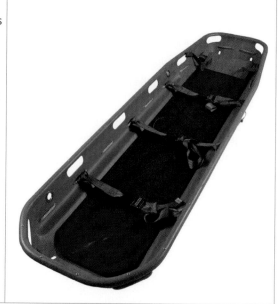

Assessment practice 3.10   (EC) 10.6

1 Name three different types of stretcher and list the advantages of each.

2 Which type of stretcher would you use to package a casualty who was in plenty of space but whose position you did not want to disturb when moving them?

Further reading and resources

www/hse.gov.uk/pubns/indg143.pdf

www.tarn.ac.uk/Home.aspx

www.traumacare.org.uk

www.spinal.co.uk

fphc.rcsed.ac.uk/media/1765/the-pre-hospital-management-of-pelvic-fractures.pdf

www.headway.org.uk

www.britishburnassociation.org

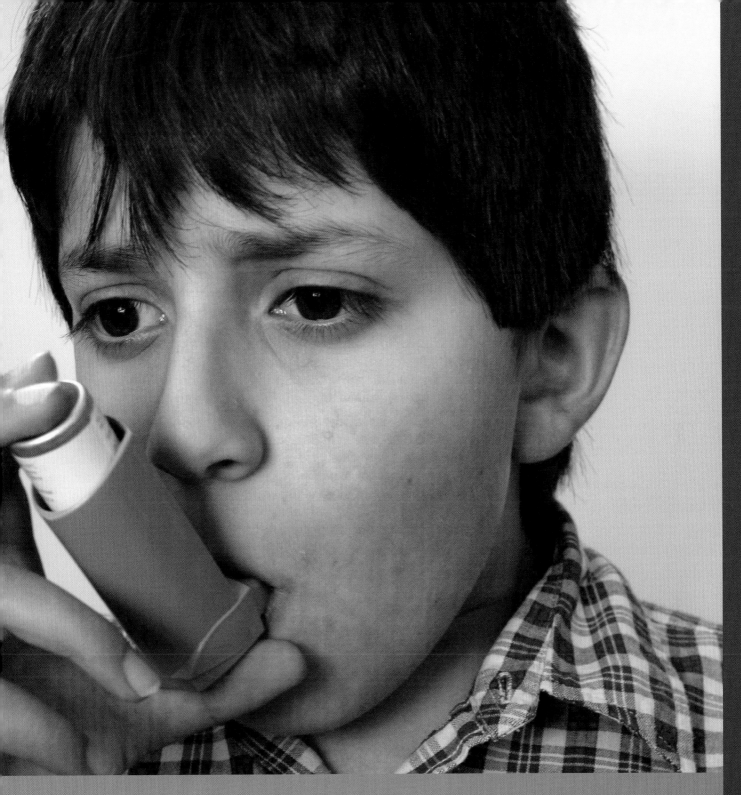

Recognising and Managing Medical Conditions for the First Responder

4

Getting to know your unit

Survival rates of casualties suffering from common medical conditions are greatly increased by early recognition, early intervention and early transport to definitive care. As a first responder you will play a key role in managing the casualty in the early stages of pre-hospital emergency care in order to preserve life, prevent further deterioration and promote the casualty's recovery.

In this unit you will learn how to recognise the vital signs and symptoms of casualties suffering from poisoning, allergic reactions and anaphylaxis, breathing difficulties, cardiac conditions, diabetic emergencies, seizures, stroke, meningitis, septicaemia and other potentially life-threatening medical conditions. You will learn how to, within your scope of practice, provide clinical management to casualties presenting with these conditions, how to handle and position the casualty to ensure they are comfortable and safe from further risk, as well as how to observe and record information required for the clinical handover to the next echelon of care.

You will develop your knowledge and understanding in a theoretical context, and in simulated environments you will practically explore the principles and associated techniques used by the first responder to recognise and manage casualties with common medical conditions. This will begin to prepare you for the final synoptic unit in which your ability to manage incidents involving casualties presenting acute common medical conditions competently will be assessed.

How you will be assessed

This unit will comprise a series of internally assessed tasks set by your centre. How they perform this assessment will vary from centre to centre. Throughout the unit there are assessment practice activities to help you work towards your assessment. Completing these will not mean that you have achieved a Pass or Fail, but that you have carried out useful research and preparation.

In order to achieve a Pass, you need to meet all the Assessment criteria. The assessment set by your centre will consist of a number of tasks designed to meet the criteria in the following below. This may include activities such as:

▶ creating a report about the recognition and management of a medical condition

▶ producing an instructional video on the use of emergency medication.

How the unit is covered: In order to ensure the content follows a logical procedural progression of care, the order in the coverage of the Learning outcomes and Assessment criteria may differ from those shown in the following tables. All LOs and ACs are, however, covered in the unit.

Unit 4 Learning outcomes and Assessment criteria (Certificate)

▶ **Table 4.1**

Learning outcome 1: Understand the recognition and management of a casualty who has been poisoned

Assessment criteria	
1.1	Describe how to recognise casualties who have been poisoned
1.2	Explain the management of a casualty who has been poisoned

Learning outcome 2: Explore the recognition and management of a casualty suffering from allergic reactions and anaphylaxis

Assessment criteria	
2.1	Compare and contrast the signs and symptoms of a casualty suffering from allergic reactions and anaphylaxis
2.2	Explain the management of casualties suffering from anaphylaxis
2.3	Demonstrate how to administer intramuscular adrenaline using a pre-filled auto-injector

Learning outcome 3: Understand the recognition and management of casualties with common respiratory conditions

Assessment criteria	
3.1	Describe how to recognise casualties suffering from four common respiratory conditions
3.2	Explain the management of casualties suffering from four common respiratory conditions
3.3	Describe how to recognise a hypoxic casualty
3.4	Explain the management of a casualty who is hypoxic

Learning outcome 4: Understand the recognition and management of casualties with suspected cardiac conditions

Assessment criteria	
4.1	Describe how to recognise casualties with suspected cardiac conditions
4.2	Explain the management of casualties suffering from suspected cardiac conditions

Learning outcome 5: Explore the recognition and management of casualties suffering from diabetic emergencies

Assessment criteria	
5.1	Describe how to recognise casualties suffering from diabetic emergencies
5.2	Explain the management of casualties suffering from diabetic emergencies
5.3	Demonstrate how to use a blood glucose meter to measure a casualty's blood glucose level

Learning outcome 6: Understand the recognition and management of a casualty having a seizure

Assessment criteria	
6.1	Describe how to recognise a casualty having a seizure
6.2	Explain the management of a casualty having a seizure

Learning outcome 7: Understand the recognition and management of a casualty suffering a suspected stroke

Assessment criteria	
7.1	Describe how to recognise a casualty suffering a suspected stroke
7.2	Explain the management of a casualty suffering a suspected stroke

Learning outcome 8: Understand the recognition and management of casualties with other potentially life-threatening medical conditions

Assessment criteria conditions	
8.1	Describe how to recognise adults, children and infants with three other potentially life-threatening medical conditions that require urgent extraction to hospital
8.2	Explain the management of a casualty with a potentially life-threatening medical condition beyond own scope of practice

Unit 4 Learning outcomes and Assessment criteria (Extended Certificate)

▶ **Table 4.2**

Learning outcome 1: Understand the recognition and management of a casualty who has been poisoned

Assessment criteria	
1.1	Describe how to recognise casualties who have been poisoned
1.2	Explain the management of a casualty who has been poisoned

Learning outcome 2: Explore the recognition and management of a casualty suffering from allergic reactions and anaphylaxis

Assessment criteria	
2.1	Compare and contrast the signs and symptoms of a casualty suffering from allergic reactions and anaphylaxis
2.2	Explain the management of casualties suffering from anaphylaxis
2.3	Demonstrate how to administer intramuscular adrenaline using a pre-filled auto-injector

Learning outcome 3: Understand the recognition and management of casualties with common respiratory conditions

Assessment criteria	
3.1	Describe how to recognise casualties suffering from four common respiratory conditions
3.2	Explain the management of casualties suffering from four common respiratory conditions
3.3	Describe how to recognise a hypoxic casualty
3.4	Explain the management of a casualty who is hypoxic

Learning outcome 4: Understand the recognition and management of casualties with suspected cardiac conditions

Assessment criteria	
4.1	Describe how to recognise casualties with suspected cardiac conditions
4.2	Explain the management of casualties suffering from suspected cardiac conditions

Learning outcome 5: Explore the recognition and management of casualties suffering from diabetic emergencies

Assessment criteria	
5.1	Describe how to recognise casualties suffering from diabetic emergencies
5.2	Explain the management of casualties suffering from diabetic emergencies
5.3	Demonstrate how to use a blood glucose meter to measure a casualty's blood glucose level

Learning outcome 6: Understand the recognition and management of a casualty having a seizure

Assessment criteria	
6.1	Describe how to recognise a casualty having a seizure
6.2	Explain the management of a casualty having a seizure

Learning outcome 7: Understand the recognition and management of a casualty suffering a suspected stroke

Assessment criteria	
7.1	Describe how to recognise a casualty suffering a suspected stroke
7.2	Explain the management of a casualty suffering a suspected stroke

Learning outcome 8: Understand the recognition and management of casualties with other potentially life-threatening medical conditions

Assessment criteria	
8.1	Describe how to recognise adults, children and infants with three other potentially life-threatening medical conditions that require urgent extraction to hospital
8.2	Explain the management of a casualty with a potentially life-threatening medical condition beyond own scope of practice

Getting started

In groups, create a table with five columns and five rows. Column headings should read:

(a) Medical condition

(b) What is it?

(c) Signs and symptoms

(d) Triggers or causes

(e) Medication.

Think of five medical conditions, one for each row. Complete as much of the table as you can to see how much is known in the group about common medical conditions.

Understand the recognition and management of casualties with common respiratory conditions

Respiratory conditions are considered medical emergencies because of their effect on the casualty's breathing and therefore their ability to provide oxygen to the body. There are a number of common medical conditions that will be covered in this section.

Asthma

Key term

Bronchioles – the small tubes that carry air in and out of the lungs.

Link

For more information on the anatomy of the lower airway, see Unit 2, page 57.

Asthma is a chronic inflammatory disease that affects the **bronchioles** of the lower airway. When the bronchioles come into contact with an asthma trigger, the muscles around the walls of the airways tighten and become narrower. The lining of the bronchioles swells and produces a sticky mucus. As the airways narrow, it becomes difficult for air to move in and out.

Triggers

A number of factors can trigger an asthma attack; most of these are airborne irritants, but other environmental or physical factors can cause or exacerbate the symptoms.

Understanding these factors can help you prevent a casualty from experiencing an attack or help relieve the symptoms by being aware of their environment or changing their behaviour. The following table describes common asthma triggers.

▶ **Table 4.3**

Animals	Furry and feathery animals are a common trigger of asthma. The allergens are found in their saliva, flakes of skin, fur and urine.
Air pollutants	Air pollutants, such as cigarette smoke and car exhaust fumes, release gases and particles into the atmosphere, which can irritate the airways.
Colds and viral infections	Colds and viral infections are very common triggers of asthma and can be almost impossible to avoid.
Emotions	Stress, depression, anxiety or even laughter can trigger asthma symptoms.
Exercise	It is a common misconception that people with asthma cannot exercise. Spontaneous exercise without warming up is the biggest trigger.

▶ **Table 4.3** continued

Food	In some cases, certain foods, including cow's milk, eggs, fish, shellfish, yeast products, nuts and some food colourings and preservatives trigger asthma.
Hormones	Some women find their asthma can be affected around puberty, before their periods, during pregnancy and during menopause.
House dust mites	Many people with asthma are sensitive to the droppings of house dust mites that live in the dust that builds up around the house in carpets, bedding, soft furnishings and soft toys.
Medicines	Aspirin and non-steroidal anti-inflammatory tablets such as ibuprofen and diclofenac, as well as beta-blockers, can trigger attacks.
Moulds and fungi	Moulds release tiny reproductive cells called spores into the air, which can trigger an asthma attack.
Pollen	Pollen is a powder-like substance produced by certain types of trees, grasses, weeds and flowers, which is released into the air and inhaled.
Weather	Cold air, a sudden change in temperature, windy or hot and humid days, and poor air quality are all known triggers for asthma.

Signs and symptoms

A casualty suffering from an asthma attack may display a range of symptoms, depending on the severity, and their treatment varies accordingly. The following table shows this.

▶ **Table 4.4**

Severity	Signs and symptoms
Moderate	▶ Wheezing ▶ Difficulty in breathing (typically difficulty in exhaling) ▶ Shortness of breath ▶ Tightness of chest ▶ Coughing ▶ Potentially **sputum** The casualty may be adopting a position that makes breathing easier, such as leaning forward, or they may look panicked.
Acute severe	Any of: ▶ Respiratory rate $\geq$ 25 breaths per minute ▶ Heart rate $>$ 110 bpm ▶ Inability to complete sentences in one breath
Life threatening	Any of: ▶ Reduced level of response ▶ Exhaustion ▶ **Cyanosis** ▶ Poor respiratory effort ▶ $SpO_2 < 92\%$

Key terms

Sputum – a mixture of saliva and mucus.

Cyanosis – a blue tinge to the lips and under the eyes that indicates reduced oxygenation.

Quick tip

$>$ Greater than

$\geq$ Equal to or greater than

$<$ Less than

$\leq$ Equal to or less than

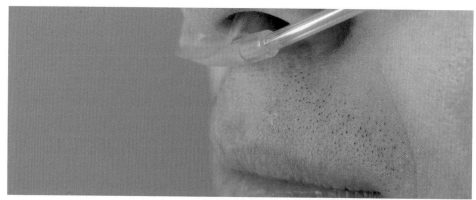

What is the cause of the blue tinge in this person's lips?

Management of asthma

1 Assess the casualty using SAMPLE to determine existing medical conditions.

2 Assess airway and breathing.
If there are any immediate issues with airway or difficulty breathing, correct them now.

Moderate asthma

3 Remove the casualty from the asthma trigger. Encourage them to use their inhaler. Increase the dose by two puffs every 2 minutes according to response, up to ten puffs.

4 Move to a calm environment and loosen any tight clothing.

5 Reassure the casualty and coach them with their breathing.

6 If the casualty is unresponsive, provide supplemental oxygen to a target of >94 per cent.

Acute severe asthma

7 If SpO_2 is below 94 per cent, provide supplemental oxygen.

8 Arrange immediate transfer to hospital.

Link

See Unit 2, page 68 for more information on the SAMPLE mnemonic and what it means.

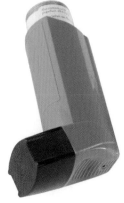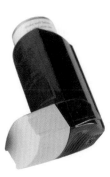

Inhalers may come in different sizes

Chronic Obstructive Pulmonary Disease

Chronic Obstructive Pulmonary Disorders (COPD) is a collection of chronic (long-term) breathing conditions such as bronchitis and emphysema. While asthma has similar symptoms (shortness of breath, wheezing and coughing), it is not considered a COPD as there are a number of subtle differences.

The following table shows the differences between asthma and COPD.

▶ **Table 4.5**

Asthma	COPD
Can develop at any age but typically in children. Many people 'outgrow' asthma.	Typically develops later in life.
A range of triggers including atmospheric pollutants but also others including cold air and exercise (see Table 4.3).	Can be aggravated by atmospheric pollutants but typically aggravated by respiratory tract infections such as pneumonia, the common cold or the flu.
Cannot be cured but can be controlled with medication.	A progressive condition that typically gets worse.

Signs and symptoms

The COPD casualty will often present signs and symptoms of illness, such as:

▶ exertional breathlessness

▶ chronic cough

▶ wheezing

▶ regular sputum production.

As COPD is a chronic condition, this is considered normal for the casualty as these are the signs and symptoms of the illness with which they live. To determine if the COPD has become exacerbated, causes for concern would be:

▶ difficulty breathing

▶ increased amount of sputum

▶ increased coughing

▶ increased wheezing

▶ chest tightness

▶ increased fatigue

▶ confusion.

Several features that would indicate a critical condition include:

▶ severe difficulty breathing

▶ fast breathing

▶ breathing through pursed lips

▶ the use of accessory muscles to breathe when resting

▶ cyanosis.

Management of COPD

6 Steps

The key feature of the management of a COPD casualty is the provision of supplemental oxygen with a target oxygen saturation of 88–92 per cent. This is a considerably lower target saturation than normal (which is at least 94 per cent). While COPD is essentially a breathing condition, high-flow oxygen can make the casualty worse.

1 Assess the casualty using SAMPLE to determine existing medical conditions.

2 Assess the casualty's airway and breathing.
- If there are any immediate issues with airway or difficulty breathing, correct them at this point.
- If the casualty is presenting severe signs, arrange immediate transportation to hospital.

3 Ask the casualty if they have an Individual Care Plan; if so, follow this for guidance.

4 If SpO_2 is below 88 per cent, provide supplemental oxygen with a target saturation of 88–92 per cent.
- 4 l/min via a 28 per cent venturi mask, or
- 1–2 l/min via a nasal cannula.

5 If the casualty does not show signs of recovery, arrange immediate transfer to hospital.

6 If saturations remain below 88 per cent, change to 5–10 l/min via a simple face mask.

Link

See Unit 2, page 97 for more information on oxygen saturation.

Link

See Unit 2, page 96 for information on the nasal cannula and details on the venturi mask.

Quick check

Describe some of the differences between the signs, symptoms, history and treatment of asthma and COPD.

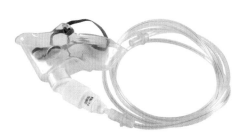

A venturi mask with tubing

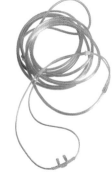

A nasal cannula

Lower respiratory tract infections

Lower respiratory tract infections (LRTIs) are short-term conditions that are caused by either bacteria or viruses. The most common LRTIs are acute bronchitis and pneumonia.

Acute bronchitis

Acute bronchitis – as opposed to chronic bronchitis (see earlier) – is a short-term inflammation of the lower airway. Chronic bronchitis tends to affect the bronchioles, whereas acute bronchitis may be limited to the larger bronchi and trachea.

Pneumonia

Pneumonia can also be a short-term condition that may be effectively treated by antibiotics. Pneumonia can be a life-threatening condition in the elderly and is the leading cause of death in children under 5 years old.

Signs and symptoms

As with other respiratory conditions, the signs and symptoms are predictable but differentiated from a simple cough or cold.

▶ persistent cough

▶ yellow or green phlegm

▶ coughing up blood

▶ high temperature

▶ fever

▶ chest pain – as a result of persistent coughing

▶ reduced SpO_2 levels.

Management of LRTIs   `3 Steps`

Management for LRTIs requires antibiotic or antiviral medication. If the casualty's breathing is compromised or their SpO_2 falls below 94 per cent:

1 Assess the casualty, if possible, using SAMPLE to gain a full casualty history.

2 Obtain oxygen saturations and correct if needed with supplemental oxygen to maintain saturations of 94 per cent or above.

3 If the casualty is an infant, child or elderly person, consider a medical emergency and transport to the nearest receiving hospital.

Hyperventilation

Hyperventilation is a common condition, usually triggered by stress but also caused by caffeine and other stimulants and some medication. Hyperventilation may be a symptom of other illnesses such as asthma.

It is defined as 'a rate of ventilation exceeding the metabolic needs and higher than that required to maintain a normal level of carbon dioxide'. In other words, the casualty is breathing more than they need to; this not only increases the amount of oxygen in their blood but also decreases the amount of carbon dioxide as the casualty is also breathing out more than the normal rate.

When the condition is psychological, caused by fear or anxiety for example, the casualty is unable to regulate their breathing, so they may continue to hyperventilate until they pass out. This is normally self-regulating but there is a potential for harm.

Link

See Unit 2, page 98 for the administration of supplemental oxygen to casualties with COPD.

Key term

Palpitations – irregular heartbeats.

Quick tip

Carpopedal spasms are an extreme version of paraesthesia (pins and needles) in the hands and feet.

Triggers

▸ stress

▸ fear

▸ anxiety

▸ stimulants

▸ existing medical conditions.

Signs and symptoms

▸ sudden difficulty breathing

▸ fast breathing despite no evidence of recent exercise or exertion

▸ paraesthesia (pins and needles) of the mouth and tingling of the extremities

▸ cramps in the hands and feet

▸ chest pain (may resemble angina)

▸ **palpitations** (irregular heart beats)

▸ feeling light-headed

▸ weakness and fatigue.

Management of hyperventilation

7 Steps

1 Assess the casualty using SAMPLE to rule out stimulants, medication or existing medical conditions.

2 Assess the casualty's SpO_2 – a hyperventilating casualty will have very high saturations.

3 If the condition is caused by psychological triggers, reassure the casualty; you may need to be firm with them.

4 Encourage the casualty to concentrate on their breathing, especially their breathing rate.

5 Encourage the casualty to breathe into their cupped hands; this forces them to inhale their recently expired air, which contains less oxygen.

6 If the casualty becomes unconscious, assess Level of Response and reassess ABCs.

7 Monitor SpO_2 and treat as for any unconscious casualty.

Hypoxia

Hypoxia is not a specific medical condition but the effect of illness, injury or environmental problems that eventually result in a lack of oxygen in the tissues.

The following table shows the possible causes and examples of hypoxia.

▶ **Table 4.6**

Cause	Examples	Mechanism
Airway problems	Choking, asphyxiation, drowning	Oxygen in the atmosphere is not able to reach the lungs.
Breathing problems	Chest injury, asthma, COPD	Damage to the lungs from illness or injury may prevent air effectively passing to and out of the lungs or oxygen passing through the alveoli into the blood stream.
Circulatory problems	Heart failure, angina, heart attack, blood loss, anaphylaxis, anaemia	A problem with the circulatory system may prevent oxygen, bound to haemoglobin (red blood cells), being transported to the tissues.
Disability	Central nervous system disorders, brain or spinal injury, drugs, medication and poisoning	A problem with the central nervous system may be caused by injury to the brain or spine or the adverse effects of drugs or medication. Central nervous system disorders may: ▶ reduce respiratory effort (the ability to breathe) ▶ affect the circulatory system by affecting the heart's ability to pump ▶ cause abnormal constriction or dilation of blood vessels impeding the ability to transport blood to the tissues.
Environment	Dust, poisons, oxygen concentrations	Being in a harmful environment may reduce the amount of oxygen able to enter the body (oxygen-depleted atmospheres), and introduce material that may affect the lungs or poisons that may affect the central nervous system.

Signs and symptoms

The signs and symptoms of hypoxia are consistent with all problems that result in a lack of oxygen reaching the tissues.

▶ reduced level of response

▶ tingeing of the extremities

▶ nausea

▶ headache

▶ breathlessness

▶ pale skin colour

▶ tachycardia – fast heart rate > 100 bpm

▶ cyanosis.

Management of hypoxia

10 Steps

1 Assess the scene to identify external causes such as atmospheric conditions, evidence of drugs, poisonings or medication.

2 Question them using SAMPLE to establish if the hypoxia is caused by an existing medical condition. If so, manage the medical conditions.

3 If the cause is identified as a recognised medical condition, treat as per guidelines.

continued on page 168

Management of hypoxia (continued)

4 If the cause is unknown, arrange transfer to hospital.

5 Assess airway and breathing.

6 Correct any airway or breathing problems immediately.

7 Manage the casualty's airway with adjuncts if the casualty is unconscious.

8 Administer high-flow oxygen for the trauma casualty, and oxygen based on SpO_2 for other casualties in line with oxygen delivery guidelines.

9 Attempt to raise oxygen saturations to at least 94 per cent.

10 If the casualty is conscious, encourage a comfortable position.

Link

For more information on the provision of supplemental oxygen, see Unit 2, page 94.

Assessment practice 4.1   (C, EC) 3.1, 3.2, 3.3, 3.4

You are called to a middle-aged casualty who is complaining of difficulty breathing. He is able to answer questions but not in complete sentences. You notice he has a blue tinge to his lips.

1 What questions would you ask to identify the cause of his breathing difficulty?

2 Would you provide supplemental oxygen to this casualty and, if so, how much?

3 What is the best position to place a conscious casualty who has difficulty breathing?

Understand the recognition and management of casualties with suspected cardiac conditions

Cardiac conditions affect the normal functioning of the heart. The two most common conditions you will deal with are angina and heart attack. Heart attack and angina are both more likely in casualties who share common lifestyles including, but not limited to:

▸ high cholesterol diets

▸ sedentary lifestyles

▸ smoking

▸ excessive alcohol.

Family history, genetics and other illnesses also increase the risk of both and can be ascertained through appropriate questioning of the casualty.

While the prevailing factors and the signs and symptoms are very similar, there are differences in both the physiology and treatment.

Angina

Angina pectoris is a narrowing of the blood vessels that supply the tissues of the heart, usually caused by **atherosclerosis**.

Stable angina

At rest, the heart of someone with stable angina is able to receive sufficient blood supply, despite the restricted blood supply, to satisfy its oxygen demand. Under strain, during periods of exertion or anxiety when the heart is working harder, the heart is no longer able to receive enough oxygenated blood to meet the increased oxygen demand. This causes the characteristic chest pain.

Unstable angina

Unstable angina (sometimes referred to as Acute Coronary Syndrome) can occur at any time but usually occurs at rest. When a deposit of fat on the blood vessel wall breaks open, a blood clot forms over the damaged fat deposit, which further restricts the blood flow to the heart. The blood clot may degenerate and may reform again, which is why unstable angina appears independent of exercise or exertion.

An episode of unstable angina can result in the blood clot or fatty deposit completely blocking the blood vessel, which would lead to a heart attack.

Heart attack

Unlike angina, which can be considered as a restriction of the blood vessels that supply the heart, a heart attack (or **myocardial infarction**) is a complete blockage of a blood vessel, starving an area of the heart of oxygen (ischaemia), which in turn causes the death of heart tissue (infarction).

How much heart tissue is affected will determine the severity of the heart attack. If enough tissue is damaged, the normal electrical activity of the heart can be affected, causing an arrhythmia (abnormal heart beat) or cardiac arrest.

Triggers

Both stable angina and heart attack are triggered by stress and exercise – the increased strain on the heart increases the heart's oxygen demand, which is deprived either due to a restriction (angina) or a blockage (heart attack). Unstable angina can occur spontaneously, even at rest.

Signs and symptoms

The signs and symptoms of stable angina, unstable angina and heart attack are similar, making it difficult to differentiate between the three.

▶ chest pain – this could be central at the front, at the back between the shoulder blades, or radiating into either arm

▶ fear/panic

▶ sweating

▶ pale skin colour

▶ difficulty breathing

> **Key terms**
>
> **Atherosclerosis** – a build-up of fatty deposits inside the blood vessels.
>
> **Myocardial infarction** – the correct term for a heart attack.

> **Link**
>
> See Unit 2, page 72 for treatment of cardiac arrest (CPR).

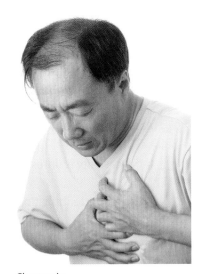

Chest pain

▶ nausea

▶ palpitations.

The following table shows the differences between stable angina and a heart attack.

▶ **Table 4.7**

Difference	Stable angina	Unstable angina	Heart attack
History	The casualty is aware of their condition as it has happened before		The casualty is unaware of an existing medical condition and/ or it has not happened before
Medication	The casualty has medication for their condition		The casualty does not have medication
Treatment	Is relieved with medication and rest	Is not relieved with medication or rest	
Prognosis	Not life threatening	Can be life threatening	Life threatening

While the casualty with unstable angina may be aware of their condition, it is not possible to differentiate between unstable angina and heart attack. It is therefore assumed that if the casualty has chest pain that is not relieved by their medication or rest, then they are having a heart attack.

Management of angina

7 Steps

1. Assess the casualty using SAMPLE to establish medication or existing medical conditions.

2. Assess the casualty's airway and breathing.

3. If the condition is known or the casualty has medication – assume angina.
   - Sit the casualty, preferably on the floor, up against a wall for support.
   - Enable the casualty to administer their medication – typically glyceryl trinitrate (GTN) delivered as an oral spray or sublingual (under the tongue) tablet that dissolves.
   - If there is no improvement after 5 minutes, administer a second dose.
   - If there is no improvement after 5 minutes, administer a third dose.
   - If there is no improvement after 5 minutes, assume unstable angina and follow heart attack protocols.

4. If the condition is not known or the casualty does not have medication – assume heart attack.
   - Enable the casualty to chew 300 mg aspirin, providing the casualty has no allergy.
   - Prepare for defibrillation and immediate transportation to hospital.

5. Assess the casualty's oxygen saturation. Administer oxygen if the saturation falls below 94 per cent.

6. If the casualty is unresponsive, provide supplemental oxygen to a target of >94 per cent.

7. Prepare for defibrillation and CPR.

Assessment practice 4.2   (C, EC) 4.1, 4.2

You are called to a casualty complaining of chest pain. She is unable to speak but is able to nod and shake her head.

1 How would you determine whether the casualty is suffering from angina or a heart attack?

2 If you suspected angina, what medication would you expect the casualty to take?

3 How would your management change if the casualty did not show signs of recovery?

Understand the recognition and management of a casualty suffering a suspected stroke

A stroke is a neurological condition caused by a reduction in oxygenated blood to the brain and can be thought of as a heart attack that affects the brain. Without an adequate supply of oxygen, brain tissue can be damaged; the size of the area affected will determine the severity. The area of the brain affected may determine the symptoms.

Cerebrovascular accident

A stroke – or cerebrovascular accident (CVA) – is in most cases caused by a clot (thrombus) forming within a blood vessel or a blockage caused by fatty deposits from elsewhere in the body, in exactly the same manner that can cause a heart attack. This type of stroke is called an **ischaemic** stroke and accounts for over 80 per cent of stroke cases. Haemorrhagic strokes are caused by a bleed from a blood vessel that feeds the brain and are less common.

A stroke can also be caused by a bleed within the brain or between the brain and the **meninges**.

Triggers

There are no triggers for a stroke but several risk factors increase an individual's likelihood of having a stroke.

- high blood pressure
- previous heart condition (especially atrial fibrillation)
- high cholesterol levels
- diabetes
- smoking
- alcohol and substance abuse
- lack of exercise.

Quick tip

Aspirin does not 'thin the blood', nor will it remove the pain of the heart attack. Aspirin is a platelet aggregation inhibitor, i.e. it prevents blood from clotting. Aspirin is given pre-emptively in case the casualty goes into cardiac arrest. When the casualty is in cardiac arrest, blood flow stops and clots may form in the blood stream. If the casualty is successfully resuscitated, these blood clots can be moved around the body where they can cause further damage. The administration of aspirin prior to cardiac arrest reduces the likelihood of clot formation.

Quick check

Why is aspirin given to casualties who are suspected of suffering from a heart attack?

Key terms

Ischaemia – inadequate blood supply to an organ or part of the body.

Meninges – the layers of tough, fibrous tissue that surround the brain and the spinal cord.

Link

See page 190 for more information on meningitis.

Signs and symptoms

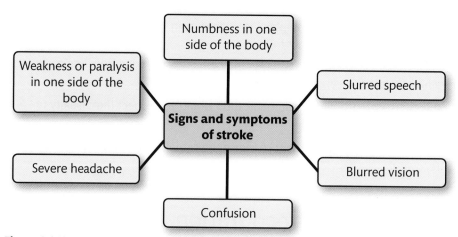

Figure 4.1 Signs and symptoms of a stroke

The FAST Test

A quick and accepted assessment of stroke should be conducted on all casualties presenting with the above signs and symptoms shown in **Figure 4.1**.

Face   Ask the casualty to smile or show their teeth. An asymmetry on the face or dropping on one side is a concern.

Arms   Hold the casualty's hands and ask them to grip yours firmly. If the casualty is unable to grip evenly with both hands, this would indicate a concern.

Speech   Slurred words, difficulty speaking, or drooling indicates a concern.

Time critical   Arrange immediate transportation to hospital.

Management of a stroke   `6 Steps`

1   Assess the casualty using SAMPLE to rule out drugs, alcohol, medication or existing medical conditions.

2   If a stroke is suspected, perform the FAST Test.

3   Assess the casualty's airway and breathing.
- Supplemental oxygen is not required unless their oxygen saturation falls below 94 per cent.

4   Check blood glucose levels as hypoglycaemia may mimic a stroke with both slurred speech and reduced level or response.

5   Record the time of the onset and any other observations on the Patient Report Form (PRF).

6   The casualty should be transported in a **semi-recumbent position**.

Transient ischaemic attack

A transient ischaemic attack (TIA) is a short-term stroke where the signs and symptoms may appear identical but the effects are short lasting, any time between a few minutes or several hours.

As the first responder you will not be able to diagnose whether the casualty is experiencing a TIA or another type of stroke, so the casualty is treated in the same way and transported to hospital. If the signs and symptoms have passed by the time you arrive, the casualty should still transported to hospital as a TIA can sometimes be a precursor to a full stroke. The casualty will still need to be assessed professionally by the next echelon of care.

Assessment practice 4.3	(C, EC) 7.1, 7.2

You are called to a casualty who presents with a reduced level of response and slurred speech. They appear confused. You think the casualty may be suffering a stroke.

1 How would you confirm this?

2 What other causes could be responsible for the casualty's signs and symptoms?

Explore the recognition and management of a casualty suffering from allergic reactions and anaphylaxis

Allergic reactions, including the most extreme form, anaphylactic shock, occur because the body's immune system reacts inappropriately in response to the presence of a substance that it perceives as a threat.

On exposure to an allergen, the casualty's antibodies cause the sudden release of chemical substances, including **histamine**, from cells in the blood and tissues where they are stored. The effects of this reaction will manifest as a mild, moderate or anaphylactic reaction.

Mild allergic reactions

The most common forms of allergic reaction are limited to specific parts of the body, typically **hives** at the point of contact, but also itchy or watery eyes, and nasal congestion. Mild allergic reactions may cause swelling around the lips and eyes.

Moderate allergic reactions

If the signs and symptoms spread to other parts of the body, such as whole-body hives, it is considered to be a moderate allergic reaction.

Anaphylaxis

Anaphylaxis is an extreme and severe allergic reaction. The whole body is affected, often within minutes of exposure to the allergen but sometimes after hours.

Link

See page 181 for more information on hypoglycaemia.

Key term

Semi-recumbent position – sitting at an angle of about 45 degrees.

Quick tip

Aspirin should not be given when managing a stroke. The anti-coagulation properties required in cardiac arrest are of no benefit in a stroke situation and will exacerbate the condition if it is haemorrhagic.

Quick check

1 What does FAST stand for?

2 How would you test to see if the casualty is 'Fast Positive'?

Key terms

Histamine – a compound that is released by cells in response to injury, and in allergic and inflammatory reactions, causing the contraction of smooth muscle and dilation of capillaries.

Hives – a raised, itchy rash.

After an initial exposure or 'sensitising dose' to a substance like bee-sting toxin at some point in the person's life, their immune system becomes sensitised to that allergen. On a subsequent exposure or 'shocking dose', an allergic reaction occurs when the casualty's body produces an excessive amount of histamines.

This mechanism is so sensitive that minute quantities of the allergen can cause a reaction, such as rashes appearing, difficulty breathing or vomiting. An over-production of histamines increases the permeability of the blood vessel walls and a further increase causes fluid to leak from the blood vessels into the cells of the tissues, causing characteristic swelling (especially visible around the mucous membranes of the eyes and mouth) and potentially a serious reduction of blood pressure. In asthmatics, the effect is mainly on the lungs.

In the United Kingdom, mortality rates for anaphylaxis have been reported as up to 0.05 per 100 000 population, or around 10–20 a year.

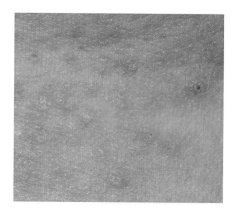

An allergic rash

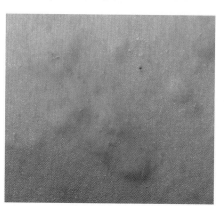

Hives – a severe allergic reaction

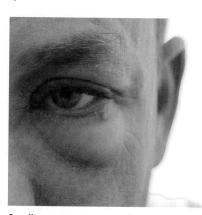

Swollen eyes are a sign of an allergic reaction

Triggers

The triggers to allergic reactions may appear random and disparate but the commonality is that they are all proteins.

▶ **Table 4.8**

Triggers	Examples
Nuts	Peanuts, tree nuts (e.g. almonds, walnuts, cashews, Brazils), sesame seeds
Seafood and shellfish	Fish, crab, lobster, prawns, oysters
Venom	Wasp, bee or jellyfish stings, snake bites
Medication	Penicillin, morphine
Latex	Gloves, condoms
Dairy products	Milk, yoghurt, cheese, eggs

Management of mild and moderate allergic reactions

Assess the casualty using SAMPLE to establish medication or existing medical conditions.

Mild allergic reactions

Mild allergic reactions are typically managed successfully with topical or oral antihistamines and require no further treatment.

Moderate allergic reactions

If the person has had a moderate reaction with only skin symptoms, adrenaline may not be necessary and they may just need their antihistamines. The allergen should be removed if possible.

The casualty should be sitting down, leaning against a wall, in order to:

▶ promote fluid drainage from the upper airway

▶ increase blood pressure

▶ ease breathing

▶ reduce oxygen demand.

If the casualty is feeling faint or dizzy they should lie down with their feet raised, as a cardiac arrest may follow.

Management of anaphylaxis
7 Steps

1 An adrenaline injection must be given as soon as anaphylaxis is suspected. If the person is carrying an adrenaline injection pen, they may be able to inject themselves or you can help them to use it.

2 If an ambulance has not been called, it should be done at this point.

3 If there is no improvement within 5 minutes, a second injection may be needed until the condition improves. Recovery normally occurs fairly quickly once adrenaline has been received.

4 If the casualty is unconscious, check their airways are open and clear and check their breathing.

5 If they are breathing, maintain the airway and continually monitor it.

6 Provide high-flow oxygen.

7 If the casualty's breathing stops, commence CPR.

The use of adrenaline via auto-injector

Adrenaline is available in pre-filled auto-injectors and is used for severe or anaphylactic allergic reactions. The responder may assist the casualty to take their own medication or may administer the medication if the casualty is unable to.

Adrenaline auto-injectors are typically available in the following doses:

▶ Adult – 0.3 mg in 1 : 1000 solution

▶ Child – 0.15 mg in 1 : 1000 solution.

Using an auto-injector

1 Check to ensure the auto-injector:
- is adrenaline for the management of anaphylaxis
- belongs to the casualty
- is in date
- is the appropriate dose for the casualty – child or adult.

2 Identify the end from which the needle is deployed.

3 Remove the safety cap from the other end.

4 The injection site is the upper, outer quarter of the thigh.
- The auto-injector can be used through clothing but ensure there is nothing in pockets around the area you are about to inject, or that you insert it through clothing seams as the needle may not pierce the skin.

5 Gripping the auto-injector, press it firmly into the casualty's thigh and hold it in place for at least 10 seconds to ensure all of the adrenaline has been administered.

6 Rub the area to ensure dispersal of the adrenaline in the muscle tissue.

7 Dispose of the auto-injector appropriately.

8 Monitor the casualty's vital signs.

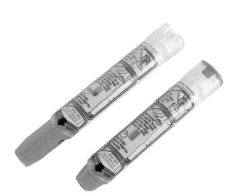

Used and unused auto-injectors

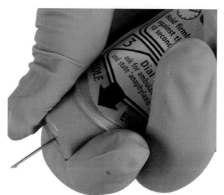

Auto-injector with needle deployed

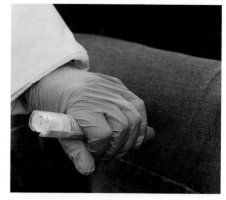

Hold the auto-injector against the casualty's upper outer thigh

The use of adrenaline auto-injectors under Group Protocols

In some cases you may be provided with certain drugs for use within your role. While it is not within your remit to prescribe medications, organisations may have Group Protocols written by a Registered Healthcare Professional that allow members of the organisation to administer certain drugs in specific situations. Adrenaline in the form of a single dose auto-injector may be one such drug provided to you.

Administer an auto-injector you carry in case of anaphylactic emergency as soon as possible to the casualty.

After use, you must:

▶ record the time the first and subsequent doses were given on the PRF

▶ notify your employer that adrenaline has been administered to the casualty

▶ dispose of the auto-injector in a sharps bin

▶ re-stock the equipment bag with the correct number of adrenaline auto-injectors as directed by the Group Protocols.

> **Quick check**
>
> What checks should be made before administering adrenaline via an auto-injector?

Assessment practice 4.4 (C, EC) 2.1, 2.2

You are in a restaurant when a customer clutches their throat and looks panicked. You ask 'Are you choking?' and they shake their head.

1 What would your first actions be for this casualty?

2 In this environment, how many triggers to an allergic reaction can you think of?

3 How would you differentiate between a mild, moderate or anaphylactic allergy?

Understand the recognition and management of a casualty having a seizure

Seizures are typically used to describe the uncontrolled shaking or violent jerking movement of the casualty – also referred to as convulsions or 'fits'. Seizures can also manifest as a vacant staring or complete and spontaneous muscle relaxation (known as absence seizures).

While the exact cause of seizures is still unknown, it is known that it is due to random or chaotic brain activity and the region of the brain affected will determine how the seizure manifests.

> **Link**
>
> See Unit 2, page 71 for more on Basic Life Support (BLS).

Causes

The most common cause of seizures is epilepsy – with an estimated 500 000 cases in the UK and over 60 million globally – but seizures can be brought on by other causes, for example:

▶ alcohol and substance misuse

▶ meningitis

▶ head injury

▶ hypoglycaemia

▶ fever (febrile convulsions)

▶ exhaustion

▶ stroke

▶ diabetes

▶ eclampsia – a disorder in pregnancy resulting in extremely high blood pressure.

> **Link**
>
> See page 180 for more information on diabetes, page 190 for meningitis and page 171 for strokes.

See Unit 2, page 91 for information on nasopharyngeal airway.

Key term

Status epilepticus – a dangerous condition in which either an epileptic seizure lasts longer than 30 minutes or the seizures follow one another without recovery of consciousness between them.

Link

See Unit 2, page 91 for information on nasopharyngeal airway.

Link

For more information on ABC, see page 42.

Approximately 1 in 20 people will experience a seizure of some degree but having a seizure does not mean the casualty has epilepsy. Epilepsy is a diagnosed condition and care should be taken to avoid referring to the casualty as 'epileptic' unless their condition has been diagnosed.

Signs and symptoms

As the signs and symptoms are determined by both the location of the origin within the brain and the area of the brain affected, the signs and symptoms are broad.

▶ **Table 4.9**

Signs	Symptoms
▶ Muscle twitching limited to one area of the body	▶ An 'aura' – a feeling in some casualties that something is 'not right'
▶ Full body convulsions	▶ Blurred vision
▶ Difficulty speaking	▶ Confusion/disorientation
▶ Appearing vacant	▶ Unconsciousness
▶ Incontinence	

Some absence seizures can last only a few seconds or a few minutes, and some partial seizures may manifest as subtle twitching. Most convulsive seizures resolve on their own after 10 minutes but a seizure that lasts longer than 5 minutes is considered a medical emergency.

Following the seizure, the casualty may experience a 'post-ictal' recovery period. During this time the casualty may remain unconscious (but not in seizure) or may appear confused, aggressive or be extremely tired.

Management of a seizure

`10 Steps`

The management depends upon whether the casualty is known to have epilepsy or not. If the casualty is not known to have epilepsy, it is assumed that the seizure is the result of an underlying problem that must be managed as the casualty could otherwise easily deteriorate. A casualty with epilepsy is likely to have a personal treatment plan and medication to control and treat their seizure.

1 Assess the scene to ensure you and the casualty are free from danger.

2 Determine whether the casualty is known to suffer from epilepsy by anyone at the scene or from evidence within their pockets (awareness cards or medication).

3 If the casualty is known to suffer from epilepsy, they may have their own personalised care plan, which should be followed during and after the seizure.

4 Known epileptics who make a full recovery are not at risk and do not need to be transferred to hospital as long as they can be supervised. In these instances:
- measure and record the casualty's vital signs with an explanation given to the casualty
- advise the casualty or carer to contact their GP if they feel unwell or to call 999 in the event of a further seizure
- document the decision not to transfer to hospital on the Patient Report Form and obtain a signature from the casualty or their carer
- provide an information sheet if available.

continued on page 179

Management of a seizure (*continued*)

5 If the casualty is experiencing a seizure:
- if possible remove objects near the casualty or move the casualty to a wider area if safe to do so; while the seizure itself is not normally immediately life threatening, the casualty may injure themselves during the seizure
- **do not** force their airway open or restrain them in any way; allow the seizure to end
  - consider a nasopharyngeal airway
  - administer high-flow oxygen until a reliable saturations reading can be taken
- record the time the seizure started
- remove bystanders to preserve dignity
- obtain an accurate history from bystanders to rule out causes, e.g. alcohol, drugs, head injury, etc. (Assume a pregnant casualty in the late stages of pregnancy has eclampsia.)

6 If the seizure has passed:
- obtain an accurate history from the casualty to rule out causes.

7 Assess ABC.
- If you are able to, assess the casualty's airway and breathing. Correct any immediately life-threatening problems.
- Provide supplemental oxygen if saturation is below 94 per cent.

8 Assess disability.
- Check all casualties of a seizure for blood glucose to identify and treat hypoglycaemia.
- Arrange immediate transfer to hospital if:
  - it is the casualty's first seizure
  - the seizure lasts longer than 5 minutes
  - the casualty has hypoxia
  - the casualty has eclampsia
  - the casualty has a head injury.

9 Expose and check for injuries if the seizure has passed.
- Head injuries are common from an initial fall or repetitive movements.
- The casualty may have dislocated their shoulder.
- They may have bitten their tongue or the inside of their cheek.

10 A casualty suffering from a seizure should be transferred to further care if:
- they are not known to have epilepsy and this is their first seizure
- a seizure lasts more than 5 minutes
- the casualty has had three seizures or more within one hour (status epilepticus)
- the casualty has signs of hypoxia despite management.

Link

For more on blood glucose, see page 182.

Quick check

Why is it important to time the seizure?

Key terms

Insulin – a hormone created in the pancreas.

Glycogen – glucose that serves as energy storage.

Glucagon – an enzyme which converts stored glycogen back into glucose that can then be used again.

Assessment practice 4.5   (C, EC) 6.1, 6.2

You are called to a casualty who is known to suffer from epilepsy. They are experiencing violent convulsions.

1 What is the first thing you would you do for this casualty?

2 How would your management differ if they were not known to suffer from epilepsy?

Explore the recognition and management of casualties suffering from diabetic emergencies

In a healthy person the digestive system breaks down complex carbohydrates into glucose, the simplest form of sugar. All cells in the body require glucose (as well as oxygen), which is metabolised to create energy and allow the cells to function.

Glucose that is released during the digestive process passes into the blood stream but cannot pass into the cells unless it is bound to insulin. Excess glucose, bound to **insulin**, is transported to the liver and stored there as **glycogen**. When blood sugar levels fall, the pancreas releases **glucagon**.

This system of utilising glucose through the production of insulin, storing excess glucose as glycogen and the release of glucagon to release that stored energy back into the system as glucose enables us to regulate our blood sugar levels.

Diabetes mellitus is a medical condition that affects the ability to produce insulin and therefore regulate blood sugar levels.

Type 1 diabetes

▶ Individuals with type 1 diabetes do not produce insulin, so they have to regularly inject insulin to metabolise glucose and regulate their blood sugar levels.

▶ This type of diabetes typically develops in children but can occur later in life.

▶ The condition is also known as insulin dependent diabetes mellitus (IDDM).

Type 2 diabetes

▶ The casualty either does not produce enough insulin or the insulin they produce is not effective.

▶ This condition typically appears later in life.

▶ This condition can be controlled with diet, exercise and other non-insulin medications to stimulate the production of insulin.

If not managed correctly, either type of diabetes can lead to blood sugar levels that are either too high (hyperglycaemia) or too low (hypoglycaemia).

Triggers

Both hyperglycaemia and hypoglycaemia will be triggered by recent actions or events. Ask the casualty what they have recently eaten or what activities they have undertaken.

▶ **Table 4.10**

Trigger	Hyperglycaemia	Hypoglycaemia
Food	Too much food	Not enough food
Exercise	Too little activity for the food they have consumed or medication they have taken	Too much activity for the food they have consumed or the medication they have taken
Medication	Too little insulin	Too much insulin

Signs and symptoms

A casualty with diabetes is at risk of either hyperglycaemia or hypoglycaemia but hypoglycaemia is the most likely condition you will encounter. Diabetics will measure their blood glucose several times throughout the day to determine if their blood sugar levels are too high or too low and they will adjust it accordingly, typically by eating something suitable or injecting insulin.

Hyperglycaemia takes a long time to develop. An individual with diabetes who is managing their condition well will notice an increase in blood sugar levels before it becomes a problem and will adjust accordingly.

Conversely, hypoglycaemia can occur relatively quickly, before they have had time to check their blood sugar levels.

▶ **Table 4.11**

Signs and symptoms	Hyperglycaemia	Hypoglycaemia
History	▶ Missed or insufficient medication ▶ Excessive food or sugar consumption	▶ Missed meals ▶ High levels of activity ▶ Too much insulin
Onset	▶ Gradual	▶ Fast
Symptoms	▶ Thirst or hunger ▶ Nausea ▶ Excessive urination ▶ Symptoms of dehydration	▶ Hunger ▶ Shaking ▶ Palpitations
Response	▶ Reduced level of response ▶ Aggressive ▶ Confusion	
Breathing	▶ Rapid and deep breathing ▶ Possible sweet-smelling breath	▶ Normal to rapid breathing
Circulation	▶ Rapid, weak pulse ▶ Warm, dry skin	▶ Rapid, weak pulse ▶ Cool, clammy skin

Obtaining an accurate history may be difficult if the casualty is not compliant – a typical symptom of both hyperglycaemia and hypoglycaemia. The signs and symptoms of both may be subtle and difficult to detect. The definitive method of ascertaining whether the casualty is hyperglycaemic or hypoglycaemic is by measuring their blood sugar levels.

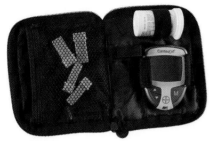

A blood glucose meter kit

Blood sugar levels

Blood sugar levels can be measured (if the casualty is willing) with a blood glucose meter. A drop of blood is obtained from the casualty's finger and placed on a testing strip that is inserted into the meter. The blood glucose meter will display the casualty's blood glucose levels as a measurement of millimoles of sugar per litre of blood. Normal blood sugar levels in a healthy person are 3.0–5.6 mmol/l.

Measuring blood glucose levels

7 Steps

1 With gloved hands, clean the casualty's fingertip with a sterile wipe. Allow the finger to dry.

2 Turn on the blood glucose meter.

3 Insert a new test strip.

4 Prick the casualty's finger with a sterile lancet supplied with the blood glucose meter.

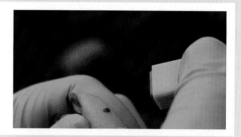

5 Bring the blood glucose meter (with test strip) to the casualty's hand and place a drop of blood on the end of the test strip.

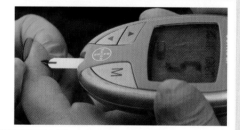

6 The meter will display a value in mmol/l.

7 Record the value and determine if the casualty is hyperglycaemic or hypoglycaemic.

▶ **Table 4.12**

Casualty	Hypoglycaemia	Hyperglycaemia
Adult	<4.0 mmol/l	>7.0 mmol/l when fasting
Child – diabetic	<4.0 mmol/l	>11.0 mmol within two hours of food
Child – non-diabetic	<3.0 mmol/l	

Management of blood sugar levels

1 Assess the casualty using SAMPLE to rule out stimulants, medication or existing medical conditions.

2 Assess airway and breathing.

3 Look for medical alerts, identification cards or medication.

4 Measure the casualty's blood glucose levels.

Hypoglycaemia

MILD: If the casualty is conscious, orientated and able to swallow:

1 Administer 15–20 g of fast-acting carbohydrates (sugary drink or glucose gel – chocolate is not advised as, although sugary, it does not release glucose quickly).

2 Reassess blood glucose after 10 minutes.

3 If blood glucose has not risen to at least 5.0 mmol/l, repeat treatment up to three times.

4 Refer to care pathway below.

MODERATE: If the casualty has a reduced level of response or is aggressive but able to swallow:

1 Administer one or two tubes of glucose gel.

2 Reassess blood glucose after 10 minutes.

3 If blood glucose has not risen to at least 5.0 mmol/l or there is an increase in level of response, repeat treatment up to three times.

4 Refer to the following diabetes care pathway table.

SEVERE: If the casualty is unresponsive:

1 Arrange immediate transfer to hospital.

2 Do not administer anything by mouth.

3 Monitor the casualty throughout.

Hyperglycaemia

▶ There is no pre-hospital care for the hyperglycaemic casualty, so arrange immediate transfer to hospital.

▶ Administer oxygen if the casualty's oxygen saturation falls below 94 per cent.

The following table shows the diabetes care pathway.

> **Quick tip**
>
> Prick the side of the casualty's finger rather than the fingertip as the side is less sensitive and this will cause less pain.

▶ **Table 4.13**

Casualty remains at home	Casualty transferred to hospital

▶ Mild or moderate casualties who are fully recovered after treatment with a blood glucose level of >5.0 mmol/l and
  o have been able to eat and drink and
  o are in the care of a responsible adult
▶ Advise the casualty to call for help if the symptoms of hypoglycaemia recur.
▶ Ambulance services must arrange locally for a message to be forwarded to the local diabetes nurse/primary healthcare team.
▶ Leave an advice sheet.
	▶ Those who have had recurring treatment within 48 hours
	▶ Casualties taking glibenclamide (medication for Type 2 diabetes)
	▶ Those with no previous history of diabetes and who have suffered their first hypoglycaemic episode
	▶ Casualties whose blood glucose levels remain below 5.0 mmol/l after treatment
	▶ Casualties who have additional complicating factors:
	  o renal dialysis
	  o chest pain
	  o alcohol consumption
	  o difficulty breathing
	  o seizures
	  o signs of infection

Quick check

What is a normal blood sugar range for a healthy adult?

Assessment practice 4.6   (C, EC) 5.1, 5.2

You are called to a casualty who is a known diabetic. They appear confused and agitated.

1 Without the use of a blood glucose meter, how could you determine whether the casualty is suffering from hypoglycaemia or hyperglycaemia?

2 The blood glucose result displays a reading of 3.7 mmol/l. Describe the treatment you would give for the casualty while they are conscious and able to swallow.

3 After 10 minutes a further reading displays 4.8 mmol/l. What would you do now?

Understand the recognition and management of a casualty who has been poisoned

A poison is any substance that can cause harm to the body. Any substance is poisonous in sufficient quantities, including oxygen and other substances necessary for sustaining life. As well as the vast range of poisons that exist and their effect on the body, it is worth considering the route of entry as this may alert you to potential dangers to yourself as well as to how you treat the casualty.

Routes of entry

Poisons can enter the body through a number of channels.

Ingestion

Swallowing the poison is a common route; this is typically accidental rather than purposeful and can be caused by drinking an unidentified substance, for example, or by cross-contamination of a product from the casualty's fingers to their lips.

Inhalation

Some poisons are airborne, which means they may not be visible, and this presents the greatest risk to you as the first responder as you may enter a noxious environment in an attempt to rescue the casualty.

One of the most commonly inhaled poisons is carbon monoxide (CO), which is a product of combustion, so anywhere there is combustion there is the risk of carbon monoxide. In a domestic setting this could be from a heating boiler that has not been properly serviced, or in an industrial setting where there is inadequate ventilation. Carbon monoxide poisoning gives the casualty a characteristic 'cherry red' appearance but not all inhaled poisons will give any distinguishing signs and symptoms.

Injection

Where the poison has entered the body through a hole in the skin, the mechanism is called 'injection' poisoning. This could be caused by a sharps injury: accidentally cutting oneself with something sharp that is contaminated with a poison, or a needle or scalpel that has been used by someone else, which may pass on any blood-borne diseases the user has. Animal bites and stings come under this category because the skin has been broken.

As the skin offers some level of protection against poisons entering the body, poisons that have entered the body through broken skin may not otherwise present a problem if they were simply applied to the skin.

Absorption

Some poisons, such as mercury and hydrofluoric acid, can enter the body through the skin. Such dangerous poisons that can be absorbed through the skin are tightly regulated, however, and most people rarely come into contact with them.

Instilled

Instilled poisons enter the body through the mucous membrane surrounding the eyes. As this membrane is highly absorbent, poisons that would not otherwise be absorbed through the skin may enter the body in this way.

Signs and symptoms

The signs and symptoms of a poison may differ depending on the poison as well as the route into the body. Generic signs and symptoms of poisoning include:

▸ nausea/vomiting

▸ headache/dizziness

▸ reduced level of response

▸ difficulty breathing

▸ change of skin colour

▸ raised or lowered pulse.

Link

For more information on mechanism of injury, see Unit 1, page 14.

▶ **Table 4.14**

Route into body	Signs and symptoms
Ingestion	▶ Residue around the mouth ▶ Frothing at the mouth ▶ Burns to lips or tongue
Inhalation	▶ Soot or residue around the nostrils ▶ Difficulty breathing ▶ Multiple casualties without obvious mechanism of injury
Injection	▶ Puncture wound ▶ Pain ▶ Tracking – irritation that follows a blood vessel along the affected limb
Absorption	▶ Redness, a rash or burn at the site of the absorption ▶ Pain
Instilled	▶ Red, watery eyes ▶ Pain

When you approach a suspected poisoning situation as a first responder, you need to assess the scene carefully in order to protect yourself, the casualty and any bystanders.

Link

See Unit 1, page 22 for more information on PPE.

Link

See Unit 2, page 65 for more information on PEARL (**P**upils should be **E**qual **A**nd **R**eactive to **L**ight).

Link

See Unit 2, page 74 for more on assisted ventilations.

Link

See page 183 for the treatment of hypoglycaemia.

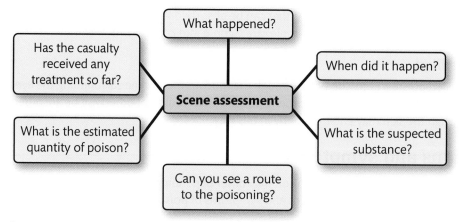

Scene assessment
- What happened?
- When did it happen?
- What is the suspected substance?
- Can you see a route to the poisoning?
- What is the estimated quantity of poison?
- Has the casualty received any treatment so far?

Figure 4.2 What questions do you need to ask yourself in a suspected poisoning situation?

Examine the area around the casualty for evidence of the poisoning, including:

▶ containers

▶ spilled substances

▶ high-risk work environments, e.g. a laboratory

▶ the activity, e.g. using cleaning products.

Inhaled poisons are difficult to detect. If, for example, you are called to a collapsed casualty who is alone in a confined space with no evidence of injury and wearing Personal Protective Equipment (PPE) such as a respirator that is around their neck but not over their nose and mouth when found, this may cause you to suspect an inhaled poison.

In the United Kingdom, legislation for the Control of Substances Hazardous to Health (COSHH) exists to protect employees in a work environment. This legislation includes regulations on how substances are stored, handled and controlled and also places responsibility on employers to hold a database of Material Safety Data Sheets (MSDS) of all products known to be harmful to health. If the casualty is known to have been poisoned in a work environment, attempt to obtain the MSDS of the product the casualty was using. If this is not possible, attempt to retain a sample of the material which should be transported with the casualty to hospital if safe to do so.

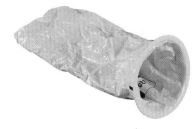

Bag to collect vomit samples

If the casualty has vomited, collect samples of the vomit for analysis in hospital if it is safe to do so. **Never induce vomiting.**

Management of casualties who have been poisoned   `8 Steps`

1 If it is safe to approach the casualty, assess their level of response.
  - Assess the casualty using SAMPLE to rule out existing medical conditions.

2 Assess airway and breathing.
  - Assess the casualty's airway, paying particular attention to any residue that may be in or around the mouth.
  - Clear and maintain an open airway.
  - Notice the rate, depth and effort of breathing and also any smells, such as alcohol.
  - If there is concern that the casualty is time critical, correct airway and breathing problems at the scene and commence transport to the nearest suitable receiving hospital.
  - Provide high-flow oxygen via a non-rebreather mask to maintain oxygen saturation of 94–98 per cent (except COPD casualties).
  - In paraquat or bleomycin poisoning, only give oxygen if saturation falls below 85 per cent and reduce or stop if saturation rises above 88 per cent.

3 Consider assisted ventilations if:
  - SpO_2 is below 90 per cent after administering high-flow oxygen for 30–60 seconds
  - respiratory rate is less than half or more than three times the normal rate
  - chest expansion is inadequate.

4 Assess all signs of circulation.

5 Check the pupils for PEARL.

  ▶ **Table 4.15**

Pupils	Possible cause
Dilated, unreactive	▶ LSD ▶ Amphetamine ▶ Tricyclic antidepressants
Constricted, unreactive	▶ Heroin ▶ Morphine ▶ Codeine

6 In cases of suspected alcohol overdose, check blood glucose as hypoglycaemia (<4 mmol/l) is a common effect.

continued on page 188

Management of casualties who have been poisoned (*continued*)

7 Expose the casualty to look for local injury or any evidence of injection, absorption or instillation. Check the eyes for evidence of eye irritation caused by an instilled poison.
   • When exposing the casualty, be aware of powders, residues and liquid on the casualty to prevent cross-contamination.

8 Arrange immediate transfer to hospital.

Quick tip

You may encounter casualties who are experiencing the effects of recreational drugs, such as cocaine, ecstasy, cannabis or LSD. Carry out some of your own research on common recreational drugs and the related symptoms that casualties may exhibit.

The following table lists several time-critical drugs.

▶ **Table 4.16**

Tricyclic antidepressants	Serious effects
▶ Amitriptyline (Tryptizol) ▶ Clomipramine (Anafranil) ▶ Dothiepin (Prothiaden) ▶ Imipramine (Tofranil)	▶ Cardiac arrhythmias ▶ Hypotension
Opiate and opioid drugs	**Serious effects**
▶ Morphine ▶ Diamorphine (heroin) ▶ Compound drugs containing an opioid drug (co-proxomol)	▶ Respiratory and cardiac depression
Beta-blockers	**Serious effects**
▶ Atenolol ▶ Sotalol ▶ Propranolol	▶ Bradycardia
Digoxin	**Serious effects**
	▶ Cardiac arrhythmias

The following table lists several common poisons and their effects.

▶ **Table 4.17**

Alcohol	
▶ Nausea ▶ Vomiting ▶ Reduced level of response ▶ Convulsions ▶ Unconsciousness	Alcohol intoxication is a common emergency, and is usually a transient problem. However, when combined with drugs in overdose, it may pose a major problem. When combined with opiate drugs or sedatives, it will further decrease the level of consciousness and increase the risk of aspiration of vomit. In combination with paracetamol it increases the risk to the liver. Remember to check the blood glucose levels especially in children and young adults who are 'drunk', as hypoglycaemia (blood glucose <4.0mmol/l) is common and requires treatment with oral glucose.

▶ **Table 4.17** continued

Carbon monoxide ▶ Reduced level of response ▶ Dizzinesss ▶ Nausea ▶ Tiredness and confusion ▶ Stomach pain ▶ Shortness of breath ▶ Difficulty breathing ▶ Unconsciousness	Carbon monoxide poisons the casualty by binding to the haemoglobin (red blood cells) before the oxygen has a chance to bind. The oxygen therefore remains, unused, in the blood and the carbon monoxide is transported around the body to the cells instead. Any casualty found unconscious or disorientated in an enclosed space, a casualty involved in a fire in a confined space, where ventilation is impaired, or a casualty near a defective boiler, should be considered at risk. The cherry-red skin colouration in carbon monoxide poisoning is, in fact, rarely seen in practice. Remove the casualty immediately from the source (and administer 100% oxygen) as carbon monoxide is displaced from haemoglobin more rapidly the higher the concentration of oxygen. This must be given continuously. SpO_2 monitoring does not work on the casualty poisoned by CO as the pulse oximeter measures bound haemoglobin, regardless of whether the haemoglobin is bound to oxygen or carbon monoxide.
Cyanide ▶ Confusion ▶ Drowsiness ▶ Reduced level of response ▶ Dizziness ▶ Headache ▶ Convulsions	▶ Cyanide poisoning requires specific treatment – seek medical advice. ▶ Provide full supportive therapy and transfer immediately to hospital. ▶ Cyanide poisoning can occur in casualties exposed to smoke in a confined space (for example a house fire) or certain industrial settings where cyanide kits should be available – the kit should be taken to hospital with the casualty.
Paracetamol and paracetamol-containing compound drugs ▶ Nausea ▶ Vomiting ▶ Malaise ▶ Right, upper quadrant abdominal pain ▶ Jaundice ▶ Confusion ▶ Drowsiness ▶ Unconsciousness	Even modest doses may induce severe liver and kidney damage. It frequently takes 24–48 hours for the effects of paracetamol damage to become apparent and urgent blood levels are required to assess the casualty's level of risk.
Tricyclic antidepressants ▶ Excitability ▶ Confusion ▶ Blurred vision ▶ Dry mouth ▶ Fever ▶ Pupil dilation ▶ Convulsions ▶ Reduced level of response ▶ Low blood pressure ▶ Respiratory depression	▶ Poisoning with these drugs may cause impaired consciousness, profound hypotension and cardiac arrhythmias. They are a common treatment for casualties who are already depressed. Newer antidepressants such as fluoxetine (Prozac) and paroxetine (Seroxat) have different effects. ▶ Monitor the casualty closely as the casualty's condition may change rapidly.

Link

See page 183 for the treatment of hypoglycaemia.

Assessment practice 4.7 (C, EC) 1.2

You are called to a collapsed casualty in a laboratory who you suspect has been poisoned. He is found unconscious and unresponsive with difficulty breathing. The casualty has vomited and bystanders have positioned him in the safe airway position before you arrive.

1 How would you manage the scene with regard to your own safety?

2 What actions would you take to treat the casualty?

3 What evidence could you gather regarding the suspected poison?

Understand the recognition and management of casualties with other potentially life-threatening medical conditions

Meningitis

The meninges are a collection of membranes that protect and surround the brain and spinal cord. The meninges are made up of three layers:

Pia mater

A delicate, impermeable membrane in direct contact with the brain.

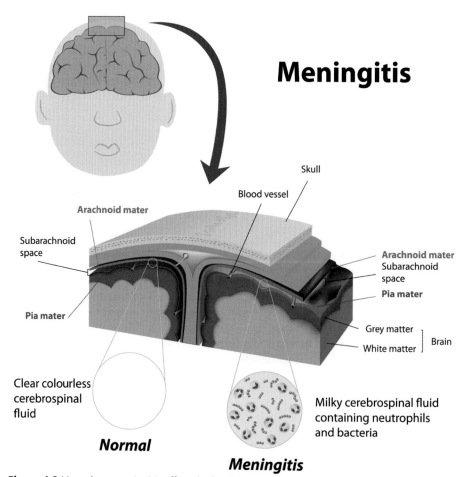

Figure 4.3 How does meningitis affect the brain?

Arachnoid mater

So called because of its cobweb-like appearance, this is a loose sac that surrounds the pia mater. Between the arachnoid mater and pia mater – the subarachnoid space – is cerebrospinal fluid.

Cerebrospinal fluid is a clear liquid that surrounds the brain and spinal cord and serves several purposes, including the regulation of intracranial pressure (pressure within the skull), shock absorption and the removal of metabolic waste.

Dura mater

A tough, fibrous layer that also binds the arachnoid mater to the inside of the skull.

Meningitis is the inflammation of the subarachnoid space and is typically caused by viruses and bacteria or occasionally by certain drugs. The most common route to infection is through the nasal cavity, where viral infection breaks down the mucous membrane and allows infection to enter the blood stream and then the cerebrospinal fluid within the subarachnoid space. The immune system releases large numbers of white blood cells into the cerebrospinal fluid, causing swelling, which in turn increases pressure on the brain.

Untreated, bacterial meningitis (meningococcal pneumococcal meningitis) is almost always fatal. Viral meningitis tends to resolve spontaneously and is rarely fatal. Meningococcal meningitis is the leading cause of death by infection in children and young adults and can kill a healthy person within hours of their first symptom.

Signs and symptoms

The signs and symptoms appear to vary dependent upon the age of the casualty.

Adults and older children

- neck stiffness
- photophobia – intolerance to light
- haemorrhagic rash – a rash caused by bleeding under the skin.

While these signs and symptoms are common and therefore their presence increases the suspicion of meningitis, they are not always apparent, so their absence should not rule out meningitis.

Younger children

- nausea
- drowsiness
- vomiting
- loss of appetite
- sore throat
- symptoms of a common cold.

The glass test

If a rash is identified, hold a glass up against the skin. A rash that remains visible through the glass would suggest meningococcal meningitis. If this is the case, arrange immediate transfer to hospital.

- A non-blanching rash is present in 40 per cent of infected children.
- Pre-alert the receiving hospital (including the casualty's age if a child) and arrange immediate transfer.

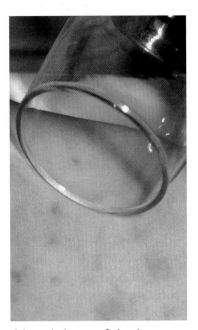

If the rash does not fade when a glass is pressed firmly against the casualty's skin, they must go to hospital as soon as possible

Management of meningitis

6 Steps

Meningococcus is not highly transferable but responders working in close proximity to infected casualties are at greater risk. Consider goggles and face mask in addition to gloves.

1 Assess the casualty using SAMPLE to rule out existing medical conditions.

2 Assess airway and breathing.
- Assess for any abnormal sounds or difficulty breathing.
- Notice increased respiratory rate and effort.
- Administer high-flow oxygen ensuring oxygen saturations of at least 94 per cent.

3 Consider assisted ventilations if:
- SpO_2 is less than 90 per cent despite high-flow supplemental oxygen
- respiratory rate is less than 10 or greater than 30
- chest expansion is inadequate.

4 Assess circulation:
- fever
- cold, mottled skin (or, on occasion, warm and red)
- reduced oxygen saturation
- increased pulse.

5 Assess disability.
- Assess blood glucose levels.
- Reassess level of response.
- Is the casualty irritable or with general malaise?

6 Expose the casualty and examine for rashes.

Quick check

What specific symptoms can an adult with meningitis present with?

Key term

Systemic – relating to or affecting the whole body. The antonym *local* is used when relating to or affecting a specific part of the body, e.g. a local infection.

Septicaemia

Septicaemia, now commonly referred to as *sepsis*, is a poisoning of the blood. It is considered a medical emergency as the infection is **systemic**, as opposed to a local infection of a wound or organ; the infection can spread throughout the body causing further infection and organ failure.

Signs and symptoms

Initial symptoms may include:

- high or low temperature
- feeling cold or shivering – regardless of body temperature
- increased heart rate > 90 bpm
- increased respiration rate > 20 breaths per minute
- feeling dizzy or faint.

As the sepsis develops, severe sepsis may cause:

▶ confusion or disorientation

▶ diarrhoea

▶ nausea and vomiting

▶ slurred speech

▶ muscle pain

▶ breathlessness

▶ reduced urine production than normal – for example, not urinating for a day

▶ cold, clammy and pale or mottled skin

▶ loss of consciousness.

Septic shock

Untreated, sepsis can either spread – eventually causing systemic organ failure – or lead to septic shock, or both.

As the body attempts to fight the infection, large numbers of cytokines are released by the immune system. Cytokines act on the cells around them and when released in large numbers cause vasodilation – the relaxation and widening of blood vessels. This action causes a drop in blood pressure (hypotension). Septic shock, along with anaphylactic shock, are both types of 'distributive shock' – oxygenated blood is available in the body and the heart is pumping but the lack of control of the blood vessels inhibits the correct distribution of blood to where it needs to be, depriving the brain and other organs of oxygen.

> **Quick check**
>
> What breathing rate would give you cause for concern in a casualty suffering with sepsis?

> **Link**
>
> See page 182 for more on blood glucose measurement.

Management of septicaemia
`5 Steps`

The casualty with sepsis requires emergency treatment, typically intravenous fluid administration and antibiotics.

1 Question the casualty using SAMPLE to ascertain a full history.

2 Assess airway and breathing.
- Assess the airway and breathing and correct life-threatening problems immediately.
- Obtain the casualty's oxygen saturation and administer high-flow oxygen with a target saturation of at least 95 per cent.

3 Consider assisted ventilations if:
- SpO_2 remains at less than 90 per cent despite high-flow oxygen
- respiratory rate is less than 10 or greater than 30.

4 Arrange immediate transfer to hospital.

5 Continue with assessment of circulation, disability and exposure of the casualty, including blood glucose measurement, as long as it does not delay the transfer to hospital.

Appendicitis

The appendix is a long (about 5–10 cm), hollow pouch located at the junction between the large and small intestines. It is only recently that its function has been understood as an important area of immune response and 'good' bacteria in the digestive system.

A blockage within the appendix – typically caused by calcified faeces, but may also be caused by gall stones or inflamed tissues – leads to increased pressure within the appendix, decreased blood flow to the tissues of the appendix and bacterial growth inside the appendix, leading to inflammation. The combination of inflammation, decreased blood flow and swelling can cause tissue damage and eventually tissue death. If untreated, the appendix can burst, introducing infection into the abdomen and leading to life-threatening sepsis.

Appendicitis can happen at any time, without an apparent trigger, but some people are more likely to develop appendicitis:

- men
- those between 10 and 19 years old
- those with a family history
- those with long-term bowel disorders.

Signs and symptoms

Appendicitis presents with the casualty having abdominal pain around their umbilicus (belly button) that, after a few hours, moves to the lower right quarter of the abdomen.

In addition, **rebound tenderness** is often noted; pain is not aggravated with the application of pressure on the abdomen but with the sudden release of that pressure.

Additional signs and symptoms may include:

- nausea and vomiting
- loss of appetite
- diarrhoea
- fever.

Many casualties do not, however, display these symptoms.

Key term

Rebound tenderness – a physical examination of the abdomen. Visually divide the abdomen into four quarters, through the navel (belly button). Press firmly on each quarter, in turn, and quickly release. Pain is not felt when pressure is applied; instead, the pain is felt when pressure is quickly removed.

Quick check

What is characteristic in the abdominal pain felt by a casualty with appendicitis?

Management of appendicitis

`5 Steps`

1 Assess the casualty using SAMPLE to rule out existing medical conditions.

2 Assess airway and breathing.
- Provide supplemental oxygen if the casualty's oxygen saturation is below 94 per cent.

3 Assess circulation.
- Note the colour and temperature of the casualty as an indication of sepsis.
- If sepsis is suspected, arrange immediate transfer to hospital.

4 Expose the casualty.
- Perform a rebound tenderness examination.

5 Facilitate transfer to hospital.

Travel-related illnesses

Travel-related illnesses such as rabies, malaria, yellow fever and typhoid present a problem in diagnosis as the signs and symptoms with which the casualty presents may be similar to those of a more familiar, common medical condition, or they may be unique.

The key to recognising any undiagnosed illness is to establish if they have travelled abroad recently. Most illness will manifest in a few days or weeks but in some illnesses, the signs and symptoms may not present for months.

Signs and symptoms

The following table shows how travel-related illnesses can affect every system of the body.

▶ **Table 4.18**

Bodily systems	Potential problems
Cardiovascular system (heart, blood vessels and blood)	▶ Blood clotting problems ▶ Sepsis ▶ Raised or lowered pulse ▶ Irregular heart rhythms ▶ High or low blood pressure
Respiratory system (airway and lungs)	▶ Difficulty breathing ▶ Persistent cough ▶ Phlegm or mucus ▶ Coughing up blood
Digestive system (mouth, oesophagus, stomach and intestines)	▶ Abdominal pain ▶ Nausea ▶ Vomiting ▶ Diarrhoea

Table 4.18 continued

Endochrine system (hormones)	▶ Anxiety ▶ Irritability ▶ Depression ▶ Confusion ▶ Nervousness ▶ Fatigue ▶ Fever ▶ Headaches ▶ Jaundice
Integumentary system (skin, hair, nails and sweat glands)	▶ Rash ▶ Sores ▶ Fever ▶ Sweating ▶ Flushed appearance
Lymphatic system (lymph glands – for the removal of waste products)	▶ Swelling – especially around the neck, armpits and groin ▶ Nausea
Musculoskeletal system (muscles, bones, cartilage, ligaments and tendons)	▶ Joint pain ▶ Muscle pain ▶ Weakness ▶ Fatigue
Nervous system (brain, spinal cord and nerves)	▶ Reduced level of response ▶ Headache ▶ Pain ▶ Abnormal sensations ▶ Loss of motor control
Renal system (kidneys, bladder, urethra)	▶ Urinary tract infections ▶ Passing blood in urine ▶ Pain when passing urine
Reproductive systems (testicles and ovaries)	▶ Pain ▶ Discharge ▶ Sexually transmitted diseases (STDs)
Vestibular system (inner ear and cerebellum – responsible for balance and spatial awareness)	▶ Loss of balance ▶ Loss of motor control

The route to infection depends upon the disease; travel-related illnesses can be caught from:

▶ direct contact with an infected person

▶ indirect contact and poor hand-washing regime

▶ poor sanitation

▶ infected foods or water

▶ animal and parasite bites

▶ airborne infections.

Management of travel-related illnesses

The management required is dependent upon the disease, which cannot be diagnosed before the casualty reaches hospital. As such, all travel-related illnesses should be treated as any other undiagnosed illnesses.

Be aware of bodily fluids or casualties with persistent or productive coughs.

1   Assess the casualty using SAMPLE to rule out existing medical conditions.

2   Assess airway and breathing.
- Assess the casualty's airway and provide supplemental oxygen if their saturation is below 94 per cent.

3   Assess circulation, noting colour, temperature, capillary refill time, pulse and SpO_2.

4   Check the casualty's blood sugar levels and motor control.

5   Expose the area.
- If the casualty is complaining of pain, expose the affected area to assess for visible signs including rashes, swellings, sores, etc.

6   Facilitate transfer to hospital.

Assessment practice 4.8   (C, EC) 8.1, 8.2

The casualty you are called to is an 18-year-old male. He is complaining of abdominal pain, nausea and fever.

1   How would SAMPLE help you assess the casualty?

2   What type of physical examination would you perform on the casualty?

3   What course of action would you take if you discovered he had recently returned from travelling abroad?

4   If you were not able to diagnose a particular medical condition, how would you treat this casualty?

Quick check

What are common causes of travel-related illnesses?

Further reading and resources

Pilberry, R. and Lethbridge, K., Ambulance Care Essentials, Brigg, United Kingdom, Class Publishing, 2015.

Association of Ambulance Chief Executives, UK Ambulance Services Clinical Practice Guidelines, Bridgwater, United Kingdom, Class Publishing, 2016.

Websites

www.anaphylaxis.org.uk
Anaphylaxis Campaign. Research and guidance on anaphylaxis and allergies.

www.asthma.org.uk
Asthma UK. Information and guidance on asthma.

www.bhf.org.uk
British Heart Foundation. Research and guidance on cardiac conditions.

www.brit-thoracic.org.uk
British Thoracic Society. Research and guidance on respiratory conditions and the use of supplemental oxygen.

www.diabetes.org.uk
Diabetes UK. Research and guidance on diabetes.

www.epilepsy.org.uk
Epilepsy Action. Advice and guidance on epilepsy.

www.hse.gov.uk
Health and Safety Executive guidance on poisoning and work-related illnesses.

www.meningitisnow.org
Meningitis Now. Research and guidance on meningitis.

nathnac.net
NaTHNaC. National Travel Health Network and Centre. Advice and guidance on travel-related illnesses.

www.resus.org.uk
Latest guidelines for UK resuscitation protocols and manual handling guidance.

www.stroke.org.uk
The Stroke Association. Research and guidance on stroke and TIA.

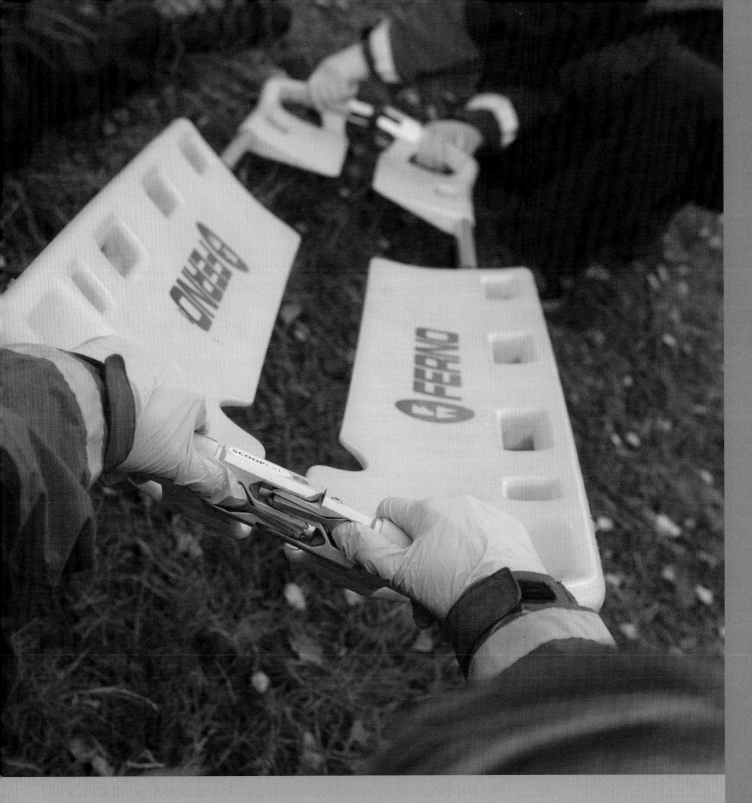

Developing the Competencies of Incident Management for the First Responder

5

Getting to know your unit

As the first responder you may be called to attend incidents involving casualties with a wide range of clinical needs, some of which could be closely associated with specific job roles that you undertake in your professional career such as major chest injuries and prolonged exposure to the extremes of temperature. However, as you will already have learned in *Unit 1: Roles and Responsibilities of the First Responder*, the role of the first responder goes beyond that of clinical management and requires you to take responsibility for the wider scope of managing incidents, including scene management and safety. When you attend such incidents you will be required to make decisions about how to manage your own and others' safety as well as how to manage the packaging and movement of casualties.

You will have already completed Units 1 to 4 in which you should have developed your knowledge and understanding of how to manage the casualty and the wider incident as the first responder, and explored a variety of skills and techniques used in order to provide appropriate management to casualties while awaiting the arrival of definitive pre-hospital care.

In this synoptic unit, you will explore and use the knowledge and understanding that you have previously developed to develop and demonstrate the skills that are essential to competently manage incidents from the point of your arrival on scene to the completion of the post-incident procedures. You will develop your confidence and competency in using your knowledge, skills and understanding in simulated environments covering a range of incidents, including casualties who have suffered a cardiac arrest, a casualty suffering with traumatic injuries, a casualty suffering from major traumatic injuries and a casualty with an acute medical condition.

How you will be assessed

This unit will be assessed internally. Your training provider will set up all assessments and they will arrange for these to be marked and results fed back directly to you. How training providers perform this assessment will vary from centre to centre. The unit comprises a series of five practical assessments for each of the learning outcomes. Two of the assessments require you to complete a Patient Report Form (PRF) as a second task.

When you are thinking about each of the assessment criteria, use the following table to help you decide how well you need to know the topic.

▶ **Table 5.1**

Conduct	Show how you would complete a task. You may find it helpful to verbalise what you are doing.
Provide	Show what you would do if the situation were real.
Assist	Under the guidance of a more qualified practitioner, help to complete a task.
Complete	Fill out a given form following an incident.
Manage	Take the lead when completing a task.

Unit 5 Learning outcomes and Assessment criteria (Certificate)

▶ **Table 5.2**

Learning outcome 1: Be able to manage an incident involving an adult casualty in cardiac arrest and assist a more qualified practitioner in the extrication of the casualty

Assessment criteria	
1.1	Conduct a scene survey and take appropriate actions to minimise risk to acceptable levels for an incident involving an adult in cardiac arrest
1.2	Provide clinical management to an adult casualty in cardiac arrest in line with current clinical guidelines and scope of practice
1.3	Provide an accurate and complete clinical handover to the next echelon of care for an adult casualty who has suffered cardiac arrest
1.4	Assist the clinician to package an adult casualty who has suffered a cardiac arrest
1.5	Assist with the movement of an adult casualty who has suffered cardiac arrest to medical assistance

Learning outcome 2: Be able to manage an incident involving a child or infant casualty in cardiac arrest

Assessment criteria	
2.1	Conduct a scene survey and take appropriate actions to minimise risk to acceptable levels for an incident involving a child or infant in cardiac arrest
2.2	Provide clinical management to a child or infant casualty in cardiac arrest in line with current clinical guidelines and scope of practice
2.3	Provide an accurate and complete clinical handover to the next echelon of care for a child or infant casualty who has suffered cardiac arrest

Learning outcome 3: Be able to manage an incident involving a single casualty with two or more types of traumatic injury

Assessment criteria	
3.1	Conduct a scene survey and take appropriate actions to minimise risk to acceptable levels for an incident involving a single casualty with two or more types of traumatic injury
3.2	Provide clinical management to a single casualty with two or more types of traumatic injury in line with current clinical guidelines and scope of practice
3.3	Accurately complete a Patient Report Form for a single casualty with two or more types of traumatic injury
3.4	Provide an accurate and complete clinical handover to the next echelon of care for a single casualty with two or more types of traumatic injury

Learning outcome 4: Be able to manage an incident involving a single casualty with two or more types of major traumatic injury and assist a more qualified practitioner in the extrication of the casualty

	Assessment criteria
4.1	Conduct a scene survey and take appropriate actions to minimise risk to acceptable levels for an incident involving a single casualty with two or more types of major traumatic injury
4.2	Provide clinical management to a single casualty with two or more types of major traumatic injuries in line with current clinical guidelines and scope of practice
4.3	Provide an accurate and complete clinical handover to the next echelon of care for a single casualty with two or more types of major traumatic injury
4.4	Assist the clinician to package a single casualty with two or more types of major traumatic injury
4.5	Assist with the movement of a single casualty with two or more types of major traumatic injury to medical assistance

Learning outcome 5: Be able to manage an incident involving a casualty with an acute medical condition

	Assessment criteria
5.1	Conduct a scene survey and take appropriate actions to minimise risk to acceptable levels for an incident involving a casualty with an acute medical condition
5.2	Provide clinical management to a casualty with an acute medical condition in line with current clinical guidelines and scope of practice
5.3	Accurately complete a Patient Report Form for a casualty with an acute medical condition
5.4	Provide an accurate and complete clinical handover to the next echelon of care for a casualty with an acute medical condition

Unit 5 Learning outcomes and Assessment criteria (Extended Certificate)

▶ Table 5.3

Learning outcome 1: Be able to manage an incident involving an adult casualty in cardiac arrest

	Assessment criteria
1.1	Conduct a scene survey and take appropriate actions to minimise risk to acceptable levels for an incident involving an adult in cardiac arrest
1.2	Provide clinical management to an adult casualty in cardiac arrest in line with current clinical guidelines and scope of practice
1.3	Provide an accurate and complete clinical handover to the next echelon of care for an adult casualty who has suffered cardiac arrest
1.4	Manage the packaging of an adult casualty who has suffered a cardiac arrest
1.5	Manage the movement of an adult casualty who has suffered cardiac arrest to medical assistance

Learning outcome 2: Be able to manage an incident involving a child or infant casualty in cardiac arrest

Assessment criteria	
2.1	Conduct a scene survey and take appropriate actions to minimise risk to acceptable levels for an incident involving a child or infant in cardiac arrest
2.2	Provide clinical management to a child or infant casualty in cardiac arrest in line with current clinical guidelines and scope of practice
2.3	Provide an accurate and complete clinical handover to the next echelon of care for a child or infant casualty who has suffered cardiac arrest

Learning outcome 3: Be able to manage an incident involving a single casualty with two or more types of traumatic injury

Assessment criteria	
3.1	Conduct a scene survey and take appropriate actions to minimise risk to acceptable levels for an incident involving a single casualty with two or more types of traumatic injury
3.2	Provide clinical management to a single casualty with two or more types of traumatic injury in line with current clinical guidelines and scope of practice
3.3	Accurately complete a Patient Report Form for a single casualty with two or more types of traumatic injury
3.4	Provide an accurate and complete clinical handover to the next echelon of care for a single casualty with two or more types of traumatic injury

Learning outcome 4: Be able to manage an incident involving a casualty with two or more types of major traumatic injury

Assessment criteria	
4.1	Conduct a scene survey and take appropriate actions to minimise risk to acceptable levels for an incident involving a single casualty with two or more types of major traumatic injury
4.2	Provide clinical management to a single casualty with two or more types of major traumatic injuries in line with current clinical guidelines and scope of practice
4.3	Provide an accurate and complete clinical handover to the next echelon of care for a single casualty with two or more types of major traumatic injury
4.4	Manage packaging of a single casualty with two or more types of major traumatic injury
4.5	Manage the movement of a single casualty with two or more types of major traumatic injury to medical assistance

Learning outcome 5: Understand the recognition and management of casualties with an acute medical condition

Assessment criteria	
5.1	Conduct a scene survey and take appropriate actions to minimise risk to acceptable levels for an incident involving a casualty with an acute medical condition
5.2	Provide clinical management to a casualty with an acute medical condition in line with current clinical guidelines and scope of practice
5.3	Accurately complete a Patient Report Form for a casualty with an acute medical condition
5.4	Provide an accurate and complete clinical handover to the next echelon of care for a casualty with an acute medical condition

Getting started

Before you start this unit, revisit Units 1–4 as you must be able to demonstrate the skills and knowledge learned from those units in order to manage an incident accurately and efficiently.

Introduction

In this synoptic unit, you will need to manage five different casualties (one from each Learning outcome) in different scenarios from arrival at the scene through to handover to the next echelon of pre-hospital care. You must complete each scenario in one session from start to finish. The start and end points of each scenario will be different and will be explained to you by your training provider before the assessment. The unit explains each element of the incident to be assessed so you know where to find the required information to ensure a successful assessment.

During at least one of these assessments you will be asked to manage a hazard as you check for scene safety.

Be able to manage an incident involving an adult casualty in cardiac arrest

During this assessment you will be asked to manage one adult casualty. Your assessor will choose one of the casualties for you to manage (shown in the following diagram). You will be expected to show how you would manage the incident from the moment you arrive on scene, your management of the casualty, and the handover, packaging and movement of the casualty. You will then be expected to complete a PRF, giving an accurate representation of events. This will form the evidence required for this assessment and must be completed from start to finish in one session as if managing an actual incident. Use the knowledge you have gained in Units 1–4 to help you to plan and practise for the assessment. Ensure you complete each of the steps in its entirety.

Link

See Principles of basic life support in Unit 2, page 71 for more information on cardiac arrest.

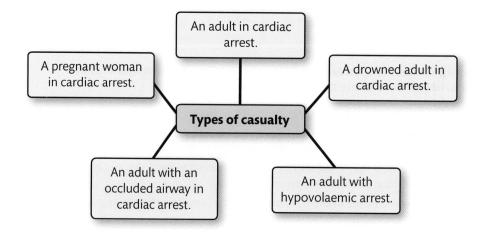

Management of the incident

During your management of the incident you will be assessed on the following six processes:

1. Scene survey and scene management

▸ Establish safety in line with the hierarchy of priority (see Unit 1, page 15).
  • Remove any hazards that you can manage within your scope of practice.

▸ Consider the impact of the environment on the management of the scene by:
  • creating space and removing obstacles
  • thinking carefully about your access to, and away from, the casualty (see page 14 for more on access and egress).

▸ Attempt to establish the cause of the cardiac arrest by:
  • thinking about the mechanism of injury (see page 14)
  • questioning bystanders about what they have seen, while simultaneously beginning management – try to establish the length of time the casualty has been in their current condition

▸ Consider triage of casualties:
  • Ensure there is only one casualty.

▸ Think about the impact of scene survey on the need for additional resources by:
  • assessing whether assistance of other emergency services is required
  • assessing the need for Personal Protective Equipment (PPE) (see page 22).

▸ Use communication equipment appropriately to summon assistance:
  • This could be radio equipment or telephone.

▸ Undertake dynamic risk assessment where appropriate to ensure safety of self, scene and casualty.

Link

See Unit 1, page 20 for information on levels of risk posed by hazards and dynamic risk assessment.

2. Management of the casualty

▸ Assess the casualty using the DRCA(c)BCDE protocol.

▸ Recognise when to summon assistance.

▸ Clinical management should be in line with current Resuscitation Council Guidelines and scope of practice as identified in Unit 2 (see page 100).

Link

See Unit 2, page 42 for more information on DRCA(c)BCDE.

3. Casualty handover

▸ On the arrival of a more qualified practitioner, you must complete a handover of the casualty using an appropriate protocol (ATMIST, ASHICE or SBAR).

▸ You should carry out the handover promptly, ensuring that all critical information is passed to the clinician.

Link

See Unit 1, pages 30–31 for details on ATMIST, ASHICE and SBAR.

4. Packaging of the casualty

▸ Use stretchers to secure and prepare casualty for transport, e.g. scoop and straps.

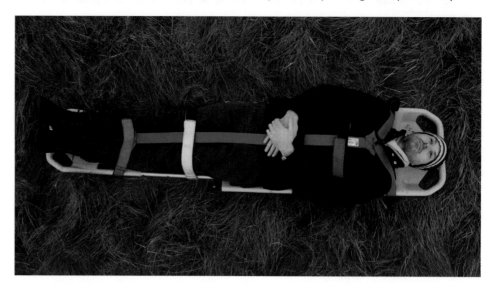

Link

See Unit 3, page 138 for more information on casualty packaging.

▸ You will be expected to be able to follow the instructions of the clinician.

Extended Certificate: You will be expected to lead a small team who will follow your instructions to package the casualty appropriately.

5. Movement of the casualty from the scene

Link

Refer to Unit 3, page 148 for guidance on manual handling.

▸ Following successful packaging of the casualty, you will be expected to form part of a team that moves the casualty to a destination (e.g. to a vehicle or to a shelter) while following the clinician's instructions.

▸ You must ensure you demonstrate good manual handling techniques throughout.

Extended Certificate: You will be expected to lead a small team who will follow your instructions to move the casualty appropriately.

Link

There is an example of a completed PRF in Unit 1, page 32.

6. Completion of Patient Report Form

▸ Following the incident, you will be expected to complete a PRF. This will form part of your assessment evidence for this unit.

▸ You must make sure that it is an accurate representation of the events.

Summary of steps for Learning outcome 1   `6 Steps`

1 Scene survey and management
  • Ensure safety.
  • Create space.
  • Establish cause.
  • Carry out triage.
  • Ask for help.
  • Stay safe.

continued on page 207

Summary of steps for Learning outcome 1 (*continued*)

2 Management of the casualty
- Apply DRCA(c)BCDE.
- Use automated external defibrillator (AED).
- CPR 30 : 2.
- If the casualty has a return of spontaneous circulation, continue to manage them.

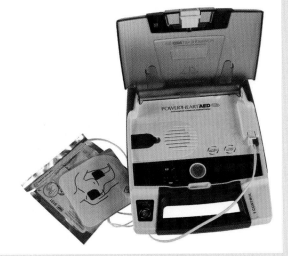

3 Handover
- Use one of the ATMIST, ASHICE or SBAR handover tools to help you.
- How many shocks have they had?
- What was the history?
- How long have you been doing CPR?

4 Package the casualty
- Either manage or assist with the packaging, depending on your level of training.
- If available, use a scoop stretcher and straps to package the casualty.

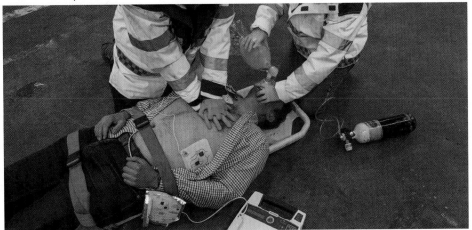

5 Move the casualty from the scene
- Use appropriate manual handling techniques.

6 Complete PRF
- Complete paperwork only once you have managed the casualty.
- Include number of shocks given, history leading up to the arrest, what you did, what you found, times recorded.

Be able to manage an incident involving a child or infant casualty in cardiac arrest

During this assessment you will be asked to manage one child or infant casualty. Your assessor will choose one of the casualties for you to manage (shown in the following diagram). You will be expected to show how you would manage the incident from the moment you arrive on scene, your management of the casualty and handover of the casualty. This will form the evidence required for this assessment and must be completed from start to finish in one session as if managing an actual incident. Use the knowledge you have gained in Units 1–4 to help you to plan and practise for the assessment. Ensure you complete each of the steps in its entirety.

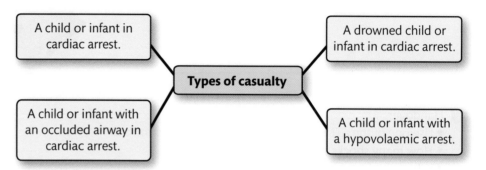

Management of the incident

During your management of the incident you will be assessed on the following three processes:

1. Scene survey and scene management

▸ Establish safety in line with the hierarchy of priority (see Unit 1, page 15).
  • Remove any hazards that you can manage within your scope of practice.

▸ Consider the impact of the environment on the management of the scene by:
  • creating space and removing obstacles
  • thinking carefully about your access to, and away from, the casualty (see page 14 for more on access and egress).

▸ Attempt to establish the cause of the cardiac arrest by:
  • thinking about the mechanism of injury (see page 14)
  • questioning bystanders about what they have seen, while simultaneously beginning management – try to establish the length of time the casualty has been in their current condition.

▸ Consider triage of casualties:
  • Ensure there is only one casualty.

▸ Think about the impact of scene survey on the need for additional resources by:
  • assessing whether assistance of other emergency services is required
  • assessing the need for PPE (see page 22).

▶ Use communication equipment appropriately to summon assistance:
- This could be radio equipment or telephone.

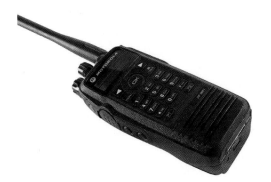

▶ Undertake dynamic risk assessment where appropriate to ensure safety of self, scene and casualty.

2. Management of the casualty

▶ Assess the casualty using the DRCA(c)BCDE protocol.

▶ Recognise when to summon assistance.

▶ Clinical management should be in line with current Resuscitation Council Guidelines and scope of practice as identified in Unit 2 (see page 100).

3. Casualty handover

▶ On the arrival of a more qualified practitioner, you must complete a handover of the casualty using an appropriate protocol (ATMIST, ASHICE or SBAR).

▶ You should carry out the handover promptly, ensuring that all critical information is passed to the clinician.

Link

See Unit 1, page 20 for information on levels of risk posed by hazards and dynamic risk assessment.

Link

See Unit 2, page 42 for more information on DRCA(c)BCDE.

Link

See Unit 1, pages 30–31 for details on ATMIST, ASHICE and SBAR.

Summary of steps for Learning outcome 2   `3 Steps`

1 Scene survey and management
- Ensure safety.
- Create space.
- Establish cause.
- Carry out triage.
- Ask for help.
- Stay safe.

2 Management of the casualty
- Apply DRCA(c)BCDE.
- Remember five initial rescue breaths.
- Use automated external defibrillator (AED).
- Carry out CPR 15 : 2.
- If the casualty has a return of spontaneous circulation, continue to manage them.

continued on page 210

3 Handover
- Use one of the ATMIST, ASHICE and SBAR handover tools to help you.
- How many shocks have they had?
- What was the history?
- How long have you been doing CPR?

Be able to manage an incident involving a single casualty with two or more types of traumatic injury

During this assessment you will be asked to manage a single casualty. Your assessor will choose at least two of the injuries for you to manage (shown in the diagram below). You will be expected to show how you would manage the incident from the moment you arrive on scene, and your management and handover of the casualty. You will then be expected to complete a PRF, giving an accurate representation of events. This will form the evidence required for this assessment and must be completed from start to finish in one session as if managing an actual incident. Use the knowledge you have gained in Units 1–4 to help you to plan and practise for the assessment. Ensure you complete each of the steps in its entirety.

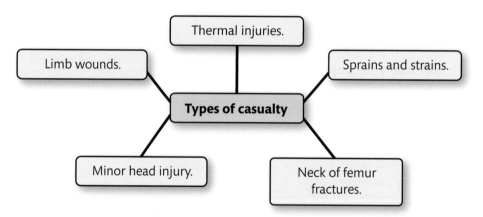

Management of the incident

During your management of the incident you will be assessed on the following four processes:

1. Scene survey and scene management

▶ Establish safety in line with the hierarchy of priority (see Unit 1, page 15).
- Remove any hazards that you can manage within your scope of practice.

▶ Consider the impact of the environment on the management of the scene by:
- creating space and removing obstacles
- thinking carefully about your access to, and away from, the casualty (see page 14 for more on access and egress).

- Attempt to establish the cause of the injury by:
  - thinking about the mechanism of injury (see page 14)
  - questioning bystanders about what they have seen, while simultaneously beginning management – try to establish the length of time the casualty has been in their current condition.

- Consider triage of casualties:
  - Ensure there is only one casualty.

- Think about the impact of scene survey on the need for additional resources by:
  - assessing whether assistance of other emergency services is required
  - assessing the need for PPE (see page 22).

- Use communication equipment appropriately to summon assistance:
  - This could be radio equipment or telephone.

- Undertake dynamic risk assessment where appropriate to ensure safety of self, scene and casualty.

2. Management of the injured casualty

- Make general observations of the casualty to help you understand what has happened. Consider the position in which you find them, whether they are moving or not and their skin colour, e.g. pale, flushed.

- Where the casualty is conscious, you must introduce yourself and establish consent.

- Assess the casualty using the DRCA(c)BCDE protocol.

- Recognise when to summon assistance.

- Continue with other appropriate assessments to ensure you have thoroughly assessed the casualty, e.g. top-to-toe assessment, clinical observations (respiration rate, **pulse oximetry**, etc.), event history, casualty history and symptoms.

- Clinical management should be in line with current Resuscitation Council Guidelines and scope of practice.

> **Link**
>
> See Unit 1, page 20 for information on levels of risk posed by hazards and dynamic risk assessment.

> **Link**
>
> See Unit 2, page 42 for more information on DRCA(c)BCDE.

> **Key term**
>
> **Pulse oximetry** – monitoring a casualty's oxygen saturation (SpO$_2$). It gives an SpO$_2$ reading for peripheral oxygen saturation.

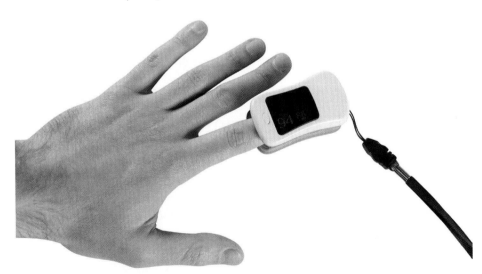

3. Casualty handover

- On the arrival of a more qualified practitioner, you must complete a handover of the casualty using an appropriate protocol (ATMIST, ASHICE or SBAR).

- Carry out this handover promptly, ensuring all critical information is passed to the clinician.

> **Link**
>
> See Unit 1, pages 30–31 for details on ATMIST, ASHICE and SBAR.

Link

Unit 1, page 32 shows an example of a completed PRF.

4. Completion of Patient Report Form

▶ Following the incident, you will be expected to complete a PRF. This will form part of your assessment evidence for this unit.

▶ You must make sure that it is an accurate representation of the events.

Summary of steps for Learning outcome 3   `4 Steps`

1 Scene survey and management
- Ensure safety.
- Create space.
- Establish mechanism of injury.
- Carry out triage.
- Ask for help.
- Stay safe.

2 Management of the casualty
- Apply DRCA(c)BCDE.
- Ask lots of questions and talk to the casualty.
- Manage any injuries found in the correct order.
- Carry out secondary survey (see Unit 2, page 42).

3 Handover
- Use one of the ATMIST, ASHICE and SBAR handover tools to help you.
- What happened?
- What have you found?
- What have you done?

4 Complete PRF
- Complete paperwork only once you have managed the casualty.
- Include what happened, what you have found and what you have done.

Be able to manage an incident involving a casualty with two or more types of major traumatic injury

During this assessment you will be asked to manage a single casualty from the choices in the diagram on page 213. Your assessor will choose at least two of the injuries for you to manage (shown in the following diagram). You will be expected to show how you would manage the incident from the moment you arrive on scene, your management of the casualty, and the handover, packaging and movement of the casualty. This will form the evidence required for this assessment and must be completed from start to finish in one session as if managing an actual incident. Use the knowledge you have gained in Units 1–4 to help you to plan and practise for the assessment. Ensure you complete each of the steps in its entirety.

Major traumatic injuries can be defined as multiple serious injuries that could result in significant physical harm or death.

For this assessment, the casualty will have at least one of the injuries shown in the diagram below.

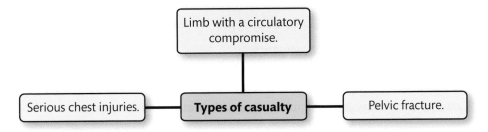

They will also have at least one of the following injuries:

▶ severe thermal injuries

▶ fractured long bones (midshaft femur, tibia, fibula, radius, ulna, humerus)

▶ major head injury

▶ spinal injuries

▶ potential catastrophic haemorrhage

▶ non-compressible haemorrhage

▶ major amputation, i.e. amputation proximal from the wrist or ankle.

Management of the incident

During your management of the incident you will be assessed on the following five processes:

1. Scene survey and scene management

▶ Establish safety in line with the hierarchy of priority (see Unit 1, page 15).
  • Remove any hazards that you can manage within your scope of practice.

▶ Consider the impact of the environment on the management of the scene by:
  • creating space and removing obstacles
  • thinking carefully about your access to, and away from, the casualty (see page 14 for more on access and egress).

▶ Attempt to establish the cause of the injury by:
  • thinking about the mechanism of injury (see page 14)
  • questioning bystanders about what they have seen, while simultaneously beginning management – try to establish the length of time the casualty has been in their current condition.

▶ Consider triage of casualties:
  • Ensure there is only one casualty.

▶ Think about the impact of scene survey on the need for additional resources by:
  • assessing whether assistance of other emergency services is required
  • assessing the need for PPE (see page 22).

▶ Use communication equipment appropriately to summon assistance:
  • This could be radio equipment or telephone.

▶ Undertake dynamic risk assessment where appropriate to ensure safety of self, scene and casualty.

Link

See Unit 1, page 20, for information on levels of risk posed by hazards, and dynamic risk assessment.

2. Management of the casualty

▸ Make general observations of the casualty to help you understand what has happened. Consider the position in which you find them, whether they are moving or not and their skin colour, e.g. pale, flushed.

▸ Where the casualty is conscious, you must introduce yourself and establish consent.

▸ Assess the casualty using the DRCA(c)BCDE protocol.

▸ Recognise when to summon assistance.

▸ Continue with other appropriate assessments to ensure you have thoroughly assessed the casualty, e.g. top-to-toe assessment, clinical observations (respiration rate, pulse oximetry, etc.), event history, casualty history and symptoms.

▸ Clinical management should be in line with current Resuscitation Council Guidelines and scope of practice.

3. Casualty handover

▸ On the arrival of a more qualified practitioner, you must complete a handover of the casualty using an appropriate protocol (ATMIST, ASHICE or SBAR).

▸ Carry out this handover promptly, ensuring that all critical information is passed to the clinician.

Link

See Unit 1, pages 30–31 for details on ATMIST, ASHICE and SBAR.

4. Packaging of the casualty

Use stretchers to secure and prepare the casualty for transport, e.g. scoop and straps.

▸ You will be expected to be able to follow the instructions of the clinician.

Link

See Unit 3, page 138 for more information on casualty packaging.

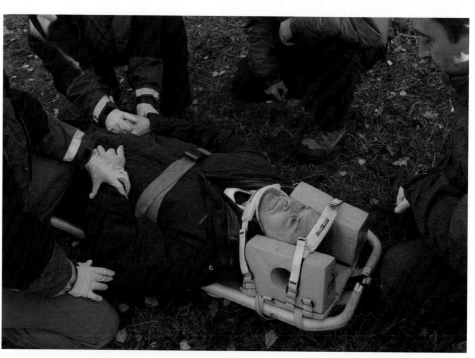

Extended Certificate: You will be expected to lead a small team who will follow your instructions to package the casualty appropriately.

5. Movement of the casualty from the scene

▶ Following successful packaging of the casualty, you will be expected to form part of a team that moves the casualty to a destination (e.g. to a vehicle, to shelter) while following the instructions of the clinician. You need to remember appropriate manual handling techniques while doing this.

Link

Refer to Unit 3, page 148 for guidance on manual handling.

Extended Certificate: You will be expected to lead a small team who will follow your instructions to move the casualty appropriately.

Summary of steps for Learning outcome 4

`5 Steps`

1 Scene survey and management
- Ensure safety.
- Create space.
- Establish mechanism of injury.
- Carry out triage.
- Ask for help.
- Stay safe.

2 Management of the casualty
- Apply DRCA(c)BCDE.
- Ask lots of questions and talk to the casualty if they are responding.
- Manage any injuries found in the correct order.
- Carry out secondary survey.
- Consider MILS.

3 Handover
- Use one of the ATMIST, ASHICE and SBAR handover tools to help you.
- What happened?
- What have you found?
- What have you done?

4 Package the casualty
- Either manage or assist with the packaging, depending on your level of training.
- If available, use a scoop stretcher and straps to package the casualty.
- Consider spinal immobilisation.

5 Move the casualty from the scene
- Use appropriate manual handling techniques.

Understand the recognition and management of casualties with an acute medical condition

During this assessment you will be asked to manage a single casualty. Your assessor will choose one of the medical conditions for you to manage (shown in the following diagram). You will be expected to show how you would manage the incident from the moment you arrive on scene, and your management and handover of the casualty. You will then be expected to complete a PRF, giving an accurate representation of events. This will form the evidence required for this assessment and must be completed from start to finish in one session as if managing an actual incident. Use the knowledge you have gained in Units 1–4 to help you to plan and practise for the assessment. Ensure you complete each of the steps in its entirety.

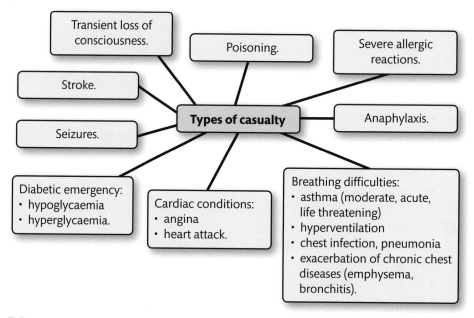

- Transient loss of consciousness.
- Poisoning.
- Severe allergic reactions.
- Stroke.
- **Types of casualty**
- Anaphylaxis.
- Seizures.
- Diabetic emergency:
  - hypoglycaemia
  - hyperglycaemia.
- Cardiac conditions:
  - angina
  - heart attack.
- Breathing difficulties:
  - asthma (moderate, acute, life threatening)
  - hyperventilation
  - chest infection, pneumonia
  - exacerbation of chronic chest diseases (emphysema, bronchitis).

Management of the incident

During your management of the incident you will be assessed on the following four processes:

1. Scene survey and scene management:

▶ Establish safety in line with the hierarchy of priority (see Unit 1, page 15).
  - Remove any hazards that you can manage within your scope of practice.

▶ Consider the impact of the environment on the management of the scene by:
  - creating space and removing obstacles
  - thinking carefully about your access to, and away from, the casualty (see page 14 for more on access and egress).

▶ Attempt to establish the history of the complaint by:
  - thinking about the mechanism of the condition
  - questioning bystanders about what they have seen, while simultaneously beginning management – try to establish the length of time the casualty has been in their current condition.

▸ Consider triage of casualties:
  • Ensure there is only one casualty.
▸ Think about the impact of scene survey on the need for additional resources by:
  • assessing whether assistance of other emergency services is required
  • assessing the need for PPE (see page 22).
▸ Use communication equipment appropriately to summon assistance:
  • This could be radio equipment or telephone.
▸ Undertake dynamic risk assessment where appropriate to ensure safety of self, scene and casualty.

Link

See Unit 1, page 20 for information on levels of risk posed by hazards and dynamic risk assessment.

2. Management of the casualty

▸ Identify any general observations of the casualty to help you piece together what has happened. Consider the position you find them in, if they are moving and their skin colour, e.g. pale, flushed.
▸ Where the casualty is conscious, you must introduce yourself and establish consent.
▸ Assess the casualty using the DRCA(c)BCDE protocol.
▸ Recognise when to summon assistance.
▸ Continue with other appropriate assessments to ensure you have thoroughly assessed the casualty, e.g. top-to-toe assessment, clinical observations (respiration rate, pulse oximetry, etc.), event history, casualty history and symptoms.
▸ Clinical management should be in line with current Resuscitation Council Guidelines and scope of practice.

3. Casualty handover

Link

See Unit 1, pages 30–31 for details on ATMIST, ASHICE and SBAR.

▸ On the arrival of a more qualified practitioner, you must complete a handover of the casualty using an appropriate protocol (ATMIST, ASHICE or SBAR).
▸ You should carry out the handover promptly, ensuring that all critical information is passed to the clinician.

4. Completion of Patient Report Form

Link

Unit 1, page 32 shows an example of a completed PRF.

▸ Following the incident, you will be expected to complete a PRF. This will form part of your assessment evidence for this unit.
▸ You must make sure that it is an accurate representation of the events.

Summary of steps for Learning outcome 5

4 Steps

1 Scene survey and management
- Ensure safety.
- Create space.
- Establish mechanism of injury.
- Carry out triage.
- Ask for help.
- Stay safe.

2 Management of the casualty
- Apply DRCA(c)BCDE.
- Ask lots of questions and talk to the casualty if they are responding.
- Manage any illness found.
- Carry out secondary survey.

3 Handover
- Use one of the ATMIST, ASHICE and SBAR handover tools to help you.
- What happened?
- What have you found?
- What have you done?

4 Complete PRF
- Complete paperwork only once you have managed the casualty.
- Include what happened, what you have found and what you have done.

Glossary

Anticoagulant: medication which helps prevent blood clots from forming, such as Warfarin.

Atherosclerosis: a build-up of fatty deposits inside the blood vessels.

Avulsion: where the skin is torn from the tissues (also known as degloving).

Bradycardia: slow heart beat below 60 bpm.

Bradyponia: slow breathing.

Bronchioles: the small tubes that carry air in and out of the lungs.

Cardiac arrest: the cessation of blood circulating around the body.

Cardiopulmonary resuscitation (CPR): the dual action of oxygenating the blood and pumping the heart to maintain circulation of oxygenated blood to the brain.

Cellular respiration: metabolic processes that take place in the cells of organisms to convert biochemical energy from nutrients into adenosine triphosphate and then release waste products.

Cognitive ability: mental functions including communication, awareness, perception, reasoning and judgement.

Crepitus: a grinding sound or feeling made by two ends of the bone rubbing together.

Cyanosis: a blue tinge to the lips and under the eyes which indicates reduced oxygenation.

Definitive care: a place where the casualty is able to have all of the treatment that they require, e.g. hospital.

Dementia: an umbrella term used to describe a range of disorders (e.g. Alzheimer's disease) which can affect the casualty's brain function. There are many types and symptoms can include memory and communication problems.

Diaphoresis: sweating.

Distal: away from. In this instance, the end of the limb. The antonym to this is 'proximal'.

Dorsum: the back of the hand.

Echelon of care: the next level of care, which can provide more qualified help for the casualty, e.g. the ambulance service.

Endocrine system: relating to hormone production and regulation.

Glucagon: an enzyme which converts stored glycogen back into glucose which can then be used again.

Glycogen: glucose that serves as energy storage.

Greater trochanter: an anatomical part of the femur connecting to the hip bone; felt on the outside of the upper part of the leg, slightly lower than the iliac crest of the pelvis.

Histamine: a compound which is released by cells in response to injury, and in allergic and inflammatory reactions, causing the contraction of smooth muscle and dilation of capillaries.

History taking: asking questions about what has happened, finding out what signs and symptoms the casualty has, asking about the casualty's past medical history and current medications.

Hives: a raised, itchy rash.

Hyperextension: where the head is forced backwards so the rear of the head moves towards the base of the neck.

Hyperflexion: where the head is forced forwards so the chin moves towards the chest.

Hypotension: low blood pressure.

Hypovolaemic shock: a lack of circulating blood volume resulting in insufficient oxygenation of the vital organs.

Hypoxia: a lack of oxygen reaching the tissues.

Insulin: a hormone created in the pancreas.

Intracranial pressure: the pressure inside the skull and therefore in the brain tissue and cerebrospinal fluid.

Ischaemia: inadequate blood supply to an organ or part of the body.

Junctional wound: a wound to the groin, armpit or neck. Bleeding from these areas are managed by wound packing, as tourniquets cannot compress these sites.

Level of response: a system to measure and record a casualty's level of consciousness based on their ability to respond to different stimuli.

Mechanism of injury: the method through which damage to skin, muscles, organs and bones occurs. This will help determine the seriousness of the injury.

Meninges: the layers of tough, fibrous tissue which surround the brain and the spinal cord.

Myocardial infarction: the correct term for a heart attack.

Nervous system: the system comprising the brain, spinal cord and nerves.

Neutral alignment: a natural position.

Occluded: blocked or obstructed.

Occluded airway: a blocked airway where no air can pass to and from the lungs.

Palpation: touching the area.

Palpitations: irregular heartbeats.

Paradoxical breathing: the chest moves inward during inhalation instead of outward.

Paraesthesia: often called 'pins and needles', a usually temporary tingling, burning or pricking sensation, often in the arms or legs. It is caused by pressure on the nerves or the blood vessels that supply the nerves.

Patient Report Form (PRF): this is a legal and confidential record about a casualty, including details such as incident date/time/location, casualty information, responder's details and physical assessment.

Perfusion: to supply with blood.

Peripheral circulation: circulation at the extremities, i.e. the hands and feet.

Pertinent negative: relevant information that would help to rule out any conditions, e.g. no vomiting, no chest pain.

Primary survey: a systematic assessment of immediately life-threatening issues.

Pulse oximetry: monitoring a casualty's oxygen saturation (SpO_2). It gives an SpO_2 reading for peripheral oxygen saturation.

Rebound tenderness: a physical examination of the abdomen. Visually divide the abdomen into four quarters, through the navel (belly button). Pain is not felt when pressure is applied; instead, the pain is felt when pressure is quickly removed.

Respiratory arrest: the cessation of breathing and the inability of the lungs to function effectively.

Secondary survey: a systematic assessment of other injuries or evidence of medical conditions.

Semi-recumbent position: sitting at an angle of about 45 degrees.

Single or double bone compartment: a single bone compartment (e.g. the upper arm or thigh) has only one bone. A double bone compartment (e.g. lower leg and lower arm) has two bones.

Soluble bag: a special bag which can be placed directly into a washing machine where the seams of the bag are destroyed by the water to allow the clothes to be washed without handling them.

Sputum: a mixture of saliva and mucus.

Status epilepticus: a dangerous condition in which either an epileptic seizure lasts longer than 30 minutes or the seizures follow one another without recovery of consciousness between them.

Syncope: fainting.

Systemic: relating to or affecting the whole body. The antonym 'local' is used when relating to or affecting a specific part of the body, e.g. a local infection.

Tachycardia: fast heart beat above 100 bpm.

Tachyponia: quick breathing.

Titrating: continuously measuring and adjusting the balance of drug dosage.

Triage: deciding the order of treatment when faced with multiple casualties or multiple injuries.

Vasoconstriction: the constriction and narrowing of blood vessels.

Vasodilation: the relaxing and opening of blood vessels.

Index

Page numbers in **bold** indicate key term definitions